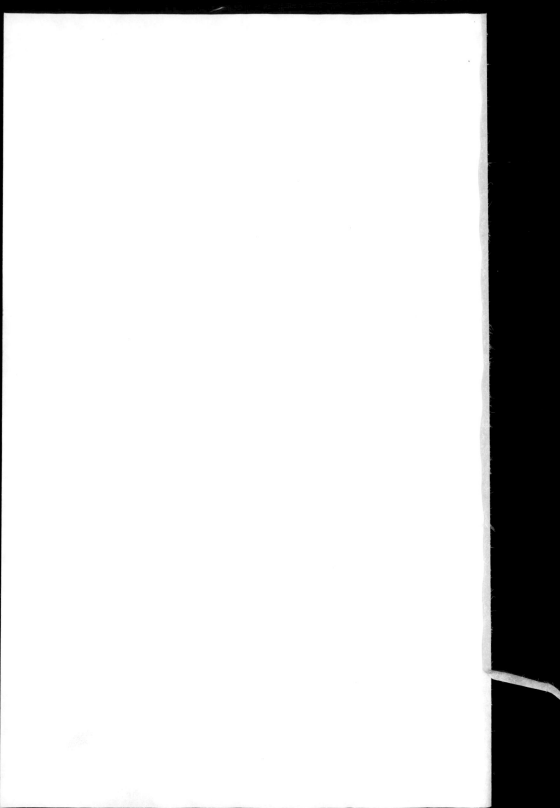

Roger's Recovery from AIDS

Roger's Recovery from AIDS

by Bob Owen

DAVAR
P.O. Box 6310
Malibu, CA 90265

The information in this book is for educational purposes only
and is not intended for diagnosing or prescribing. If the reader
uses the information to solve his own health problems, he is
prescribing for himself, which is his constitutional right, but
the authors and publisher assume no responsibility.

First Printing, September, 1987

Library of Congress Catalog Card Number 87-71065
ISBN 0-937831-01-8
Printed in the United States of America

My people
are destroyed
for lack of knowledge.
Hosea 4:6

to Roger . . .

Author's Note

This book began a long time ago. Early in my teen years I developed an interest in anatomy. After graduation from high school I took a year of nurse's training. When World War II came along, my officer training included a considerable amount of medical training. The day I shipped out for the first time with my untried gold braid, I was assigned the post of "ship's doctor."

As ship's doctor I treated everything from ordinary cuts and bruises and acute appendicitis to a terminal case of syphilitic meningitis. Then and later I experienced the extreme frustration most doctors must feel in being trained to treat only symptoms instead of root causes.

When I met Dr. Bob Smith and heard his amazing story, I realized it must be told. Although Dr. Bob has chosen to remain anonymous and his real name does not appear in the book, this story is his as much as it is mine. Actually more so. I just happened to be the one who recorded it.

From the beginning, across many months, we have been driven to seek the truth concerning the nature of disease in general, and AIDS in particular. We leave it to the readers to determine how successful we have been.

— Bob Owen
Malibu, California
September, 1987

CHAPTER ONE

Before Roger Cochran entered my life for the second time, in August of 1986, everything was turning up roses for me. But, after he walked into my West Los Angeles office, nothing was the same any more.

"Doctor Smith . . ." I looked up. Janine said, "Doctor, this is Roger Cochran. He says you know him . . ."

When I heard Roger's name my heart gave a lurch. But when I saw him I didn't recognize the man. If she hadn't told me who he was I would never have known. Roger and I are the same age and build. But the man I saw before me was a bent, emaciated, tired-looking old man.

Roger and I graduated from UCLA Medical Center together, and shortly afterward found ourselves in Viet Nam. There we served in the same unit in Saigon. I won't try to relate to you the horrors of those two years. Anyway, you've probably heard and seen more about that fiasco in U.S. history than you want.

A lot of good men couldn't handle the stress and went to pieces in Viet Nam. Roger Cochran was one of them. Having been there alongside of him, I could identify with him, and I understood. Because, for the first six months we were in Saigon we spent most of our daytime hours (and many a night) attempting to repair seriously wounded GI's that Charley had done his best to dismantle—in his most creatively sadistic manner imaginable.

The constant pressure of it all got to Roger and he turned to drugs. A lot of doctors did. As well as medics. And nurses. And GI's. The miracle is that we all didn't.

As it turned out, though, Roger was one of the lucky ones who was rehabilitated and issued an honorable discharge. After Saigon fell we were airlifted back to Vandenberg. That night we got drunk together in San Francisco. That was the last time I saw Roger Cochran until he walked into my office.

He grinned the same lopsided smile I remembered and extended his hand. "Hi, Bob . . . it's been a long time."

"Roger!" I hugged him, feeling as I did, his bony ribs and shoulder bones. "Roger," I said again, holding him away, "it *has* been a long time. It's good to see you . . ."

The lopsided grin faded and he gestured hopelessly. "Yeah," he said, slumping into a chair, "even if I'm in this condition?"

"Of course . . . of course . . ." By now the first wave of shock had subsided and I'd regained a modicum of my composure. "But, tell me what's happening in your life? What are you doing in Los Angeles? The last I heard you were in practice somewhere up in the Bay Area. Right?"

He lifted his hands as though to stem the tide of my volley of questions. "Not so fast, Bob. Give them to me one at a time."

"Okay. Sorry. But, what is happening? You *are* in

practice in San Francisco, aren't you?"

He shook his head sadly. "Not any more. I did practice up there, in San Mateo, till about six or eight months ago . . ." He shrugged. "Then I just . . . well, just pulled out."

I sensed tragedy and didn't push him. I just waited.

Roger was quiet for a long moment. He crossed and uncrossed his long legs. He took a deep breath. "You're wondering why I'm here . . . in Los Angeles . . . in your office?"

"Well, yes. Of course. But, Roger, you don't need an invitation to come to my office. You know that."

He looked around and nodded. Instead of answering directly, he said, "Looks like you've got a good practice here?"

"Reasonably so," I said. "It's taken a few years to build it up . . . but I'm happy here."

Roger acknowledged that with a nod. "Specializing in anything?" he asked.

"Nope. I'm just one of the vanishing breed. A GP. But that's okay. People like me. And I'm good at what I do."

"You always were good at what you did," Roger said without a trace of cynicism.

"Thanks," I said, wondering what he was getting at. I noted his sunken cheeks and hollow eyes. His sallow skin spoke of pain and suffering.

Roger looked at me directly. "Bob, I've come to you because I need a good doctor . . ."

"But you're a . . . but, I don't understand."

He chuckled without mirth. "Of course you don't Bob. And it's not fair to keep you hanging. Right upfront, Bob. I guess I got unlucky or something, because I've got it . . . the big one. The one that's in all the media . . ."

I wrinkled my brow in concentration. Then it began to dawn on me: the excessive loss of weight, general malaise . . . "You mean . . .?"

He nodded. "Yeah. AIDS. They tell me I've got AIDS!" He added flippantly, "You know what that is—acquired immune deficiency syndrome . . ."

I ignored the sarcasm. "I don't understand . . ."

"Neither do I. Neither does anybody else, it seems. Don't know how I got it, or even if that's what it is. But, whatever it is, Bob, it's about to finish me off. So, I came to you, old buddy."

I took a deep breath. "But, Roger. I've never seen an AIDS patient. I don't know anything about the disease, or syndrome, or whatever it is. I'm just an ordinary GP . . ."

"You're right about one thing, Bob, and you admit it. You don't know anything about AIDS. Few doctors do, but they won't admit it. They just prescribe a bunch of drugs and hope some of them will work. And all those drugs don't work. I can testify to that."

I didn't answer. I didn't know what to say.

"But you're also wrong about something, Bob. I always did say that you're the best doctor I know. The best diagnostician. The best non-specializing surgeon . . . the best with patients. And that's why I've come to you."

I became aware that Roger was speaking with an effort, and was wheezing at every breath. He gestured wearily. "One day I said to myself, I'll see if old Doctor Bob Smith can figure this thing out. So . . . here I am, Doctor. I'm in your hands. See what you can do. Okay?"

If ever I'd heard a plea for help, this was one. My R.N., Janine, was still with us, and seemed to be rooted to the spot. I could tell that she was deeply

4

moved. I nodded at her and she seemed to awaken from a trance. She handed me Roger's folder and backed slowly out of the examining room.

I gripped Roger's bony knee with my hand. "Sure, old buddy," I said, with as much enthusiasm as I could muster. "I'll put you through the hoops and see what we can do. You and I licked Viet Nam. And if we did that, we should be able to do the same with this thing called AIDS. Right?"

I could tell Roger was tiring rapidly. He nodded weakly. "Yeah, sure, Bob. Sure."

With that introduction I entered into a phase of my life that was to consume me—totally, day and night—for months.

CHAPTER TWO

As a general practicing physician, I was naturally, as
the description infers, quite *generally interested* in all
phases of medicine, but more specifically conversant
with the subjects more relevant to my practice. Which
had not, at least up until this moment, included
AIDS.

I was, of course, aware of the disease, or *syn-drome*, which seemed a more acceptable term with
some of my colleagues. And I usually read, or at least
scanned the frequent AIDS-related articles in JAMA,
the *Journal of the American Medical Association*, the
New England Journal of Medicine, the British-published *Lancet* along with other various and sundry
journals, as well as reams of the rather massive in-formative propaganda poured out by the media. So,
although I was probably no better educated concern-ing AIDS than the average American doctor, I wasn't
exactly ignorant on the subject.

But now, face-to-face with Roger Cochran, obvi-ously a very sick man, it was abundantly clear that I
had to become a *great deal* better acquainted with
AIDS immediately. I saw no purpose in trying to fool
Roger. Though he was the patient, he was also a doc-

tor. And since he'd already been diagnosed, he could certainly save me much time by sharing with me the benefits of his garnered knowledge. All this flashed through my brain in the split second after Janine left the room. Now, to put it succinctly, the ball was in my court . . .

I cleared my throat and began, "Okay, if we're going to lick this thing, we'd better get started. How do you feel?"

"Lousy, Bob. Terrible. Like somebody pulled the plug."

"Okay, let's get specific. What are your symptoms?"

Roger drew a shallow, rasping breath. "Take a look at me. I used to weigh 200 to 215. Now I'm below 150. I weighed more than this when I was in grade school . . ."

He paused and I jotted, "Drastic weight loss" on the chart. I noted that even the slight effort of talking had raised sweat globules to Roger's face. "Fever?" I asked.

He shook his head. "Sometimes. Not high. Couple of degrees. Nights I sweat. Shiver and sweat. Hard to sleep when you're shivering, y'know."

I ran down the list. Blood pressure: too high. Pulse: fast, erratic. Respiration: shallow, twice as fast as normal. Lungs: congested. Reflexes: slow.

"Bowel movements?" I asked.

"Diarrhea most of the time."

"Any pain?"

He nodded and touched the lymph glands on his neck. "Swollen a lot . . . in my groin, too . . ."

I noted all this. "And in your arm pits. Are they swollen, too?"

"Yeah, there too."

"Anything else?"

"Yeah, I'm tired all the time. Exhausted. It's an effort to get out of bed . . ."

"What are you eating?"

He grinned sadly. "Not much. And not good. Live alone . . . you knew about my wife, didn't you?" I nodded. I'd been with Roger in Saigon when he'd gotten her letter.

"When was the last time you worked?"

"February . . . March, maybe," he said wrinkling his forehead with the effort to remember. "Yeah, about mid-March. Just couldn't hack it any longer . . . hardly had enough energy to examine a patient. And that's not good for a doctor." He laughed bitterly. "So . . . I sold my share of the practice."

"Where do you live, Roger?" I asked softly.

"In San Francisco?" he asked. "Or LA?"

"Either one."

"Well, sold my house in San Francisco. Sold it to get enough money to *retire* on." Another bitter laugh. "Yeah, retire. When you can't work you've gotta retire. Y'know what I mean?"

"Yes, Roger, I know. Where do you live now?"

"Got me a cheap hotel in LA . . . just a short bus ride from your office. Knew if I stayed in the Bay Area I'd be dead before long . . ." He paused and put his head between his legs. I waited.

"Sorry," he said. "Get faint some times. Where was I? Oh, yes . . ." He flashed me a grin that was almost like the old familiar one I used to know, but it faded fast. And I saw before me again an old and tired, very frightened man.

He opened his mouth again to speak. His mouth trembled and tears came to his eyes. He wiped them away fiercely. "Bob, I don't want to die. Lord knows

9

I don't have much to live for . . . but I don't want to die. Can you help me?"

Despite myself, tears came to my own eyes. I reached out and gripped his two hands with my own. Those massive hands that I'd seen smash a dozen men in a Saigon bar were now mere bones with a thin covering of skin. "Yes, Roger . . . yes, Buddy. I'll help you. Yes, I'll help you."

The puppy-dog look of gratitude he turned on me made me ashamed of myself. Because I knew in my heart there was little I could do. Or that anybody could do. It was clear to even the least observant that my friend was dying. Suddenly I heard the words that I was thinking: *my friend is dying*! Even without a battle I had emotionally given him up like all the rest.

The anger in my voice when I spoke was directed at myself, and at the vicious killer in my friend's body. I dropped his hands. "Yes, Roger . . . I'll help you. I *will* help you! But it's not going to be easy. You know that, don't you?"

"Yeah, Bob, I know that. But I'll do all I can . . . won't be much, but I'll do that."

With that a surge of anger surfaced and I directed it at him. "What do you mean, Roger—won't be much? You've got to do more than I do! I'm going to research this thing that's gotten hold of you. And *if you don't quit on me* we'll lick it together. Understand?"

That lopsided grin again. "Yeah, Bobby. That's the spirit. We'll give it all we've got. All we've got . . ."

"Did you bring your records with you?" I asked, changing the subject. "X-rays, history, blood test, hospital records . . . all that stuff?"

He fumbled in the brief case he carried and came up with a fat manila envelope. "Sure, Doc, it's all

here. The whole shootin' match. Everything those
Army docs could locate . . . which wasn't much. But
it's yours . . ." He thrust it into my hands.

I took it, noting Roger's former San Francisco address. "Thanks, Roger. This'll save me lots of
time . . . and I don't have to tell you: we don't have
much of that to waste."

He nodded gravely, unsmiling. "Yeah, Bob, I know.
Some nights I hear the black angel flyin' around my
room." He arose to go and staggered unsteadily. I
caught him by the shoulder. He grinned a weak
thanks.

"How'd you get here?"

"Bus. Like I said, I don't live far away . . ." He
drew another raspy breath. "Your nurse's got my
phone number. You'll call me . . .? Soon?"

I nodded. "Soon." I held up the envelope. "I'm going to go through this tonight . . . make a few phone
calls . . . refresh myself on the literature. Then I'll get
back to you. Couple of days? Okay?"

"Yeah," he said and the bitterness was back in his
voice. "But don't depend too much on that stuff
you've got in your hands . . . it didn't help some of
the best Army docs to help me."

"What do you mean—don't depend on it? It's all
I've got!" A twinge of panic touched me that I hoped
didn't show on my face.

Roger straightened slowly to his full height and
when he spoke it was with the old fire. "Bob, I'm not
kidding myself. I know I can't help myself now. You
know that. And AIDS is killing me like it's killing
lots of guys. And as of now . . ."

He paused before he spoke, measuring the words.
"*As of this minute* there's nobody . . . *nobody* that's
given me or those thousands of other AIDS victims

11

hardly a ray of hope . . . not one . . ."

He grabbed the door jamb to steady himself. His blue eyes bored into mine and for a moment I saw my doctor buddy who'd worked with me on hundreds of battered GI's. "Doctor Bob Smith, you're a good doc. A lot of GI's owe their life to you. I'm one of them. Once again my life is in your hands. I'm depending upon you! I'm depending upon you to find a way to save my life!"

I thought of the night Roger had OD'ed and I'd worked with him for hours. It'd been a narrow squeak. If possible, this was even worse. I watched the fire go out of his eye and he slumped to a chair. He looked up apologetically. "Sorry, Bob . . . sorry. Guess I'd better go now. Will you have your nurse call me a cab?"

I followed as Roger hobbled down the hall to the waiting room. Janine had heard us and was on the phone. She hung up and smiled at us. "A cab will be here in five minutes," she said and took Roger Cochran's arm. Together they shuffled to the front door.

Roger didn't look back. I stood watching until the door closed.

CHAPTER THREE

The coral tree blooms were flashing scarlet in the setting sun along San Vicente Boulevard and the joggers were out in full force. But I was hardly aware of any of it. After Roger left my office that afternoon I could hardly concentrate on the few remaining patients. On the car seat beside me was Roger's fat manila envelope. I had hurriedly glanced at it before Janine brought in the next patient. After dinner I planned to hide away in my home office to read it thoroughly.

Mary met me at the door with a radiant smile. "Hi, Honey," she said, "you've just got time to shower and change . . ."

I looked at her blankly. "For what?"

"Don't tell me you've forgotten? It's our anniversary. And we've got a date. Remember? Dinner and dancing." A slight frown clouded her smile. "Bob you do remember?"

"Of course I remember," I said, sliding the tickets from my shirt pocket. "But I had quite a shock this afternoon, Honey. And I've been in a daze for the last couple of hours."

Mary hugged me warmly. "Are you alright? Would you rather not . . .?" she asked slowly.

I drew her close and kissed her. "Rather not? Don't be silly. I've been looking forward to this evening. I'll be ready in fifteen minutes."

The Los Angeles skyline was gorgeous from the Bonaventure. And the filet was charbroiled to perfection. Though I did my best to concentrate on our celebration, I often found my mind wandering. Just before dessert, Mary touched my hand. "Bob, there is something troubling you. Would you like to talk about it?"

Mary and I have tried to make it a rule never to bring discussions of my work to the dinner table. But we have made some exceptions. I sighed. "Honey, if you don't mind . . . just a little. Then I promise I'll give you my full attention."

"Of course . . . we've got plenty of time."

I touched her fingers to my lips. "I'm so fortunate—so very fortunate," I said. "And these years together have been the best I've ever lived."

Then I told her about Roger. And the AIDS. And about his impassioned plea for help.

"Can you do it, Bob? I mean, can you save his life? When all the others have failed?"

"That's what's bothering me, Honey," I admitted. "Roger and I went through med school together. And Viet Nam. And now this. I don't know if I can help him. But I do know that if I don't help him, he's going to die . . ." My voice trailed off.

Mary was looking at me with her trusting brown eyes. "Bob, I believe in you . . . and Roger believes in you." She gripped my arm with her strong fingers. "You can do it, Bob. I know you can do it. You can save his life. I know it. I just *know* you can."

14

"But the experts . . ." I began, "and the researchers . . ."

"Forget them, Honey. They're obviously on the wrong track."

"But who am I, Mary? I'm not a researcher. I'm a general practitioner. I deliver babies and treat colds. I set broken bones. I don't know how to cure AIDS . . ." I drew a long breath and just looked at her. "I don't know how to cure AIDS. I really don't know how to cure AIDS."

She looked at me soberly. "Neither does anybody else. So it might just as well be you who does it. And, *Bob, you can do it*. You can. I just know it."

It was past midnight when we got home and snuggled happily. Afterwards I clasped my hands behind my head and stared into the darkness. Beside me Mary breathed softly, her sleep untroubled. I was keenly aware that Roger's manila envelope lay on my desk untouched.

At the first buzz of my bedside phone I was fully awake. "Yes . . . five minutes apart? Be right there. Thanks."

Mary stirred slightly. "Another delivery?" Her throaty voice was heavy with sleep.

I leaned over and kissed her. "Yes, Honey. Go back to sleep. Don't know when I'll be back . . ."

"I love you," she said and was instantly asleep.

The delivery was routine, but it was 6:30 A.M. by the time I had cleaned up and showered at the hospital. Three or four other doctors were in the cafeteria when I entered. Not until that moment did I think of Roger's envelope again. I was relaxing with my second cup of coffee when Dan Halley stopped by.

"Do you mind, Bob?" he asked, indicating the other chair.

15

"Please do," I said, sliding my tray over. Halley is an internist and we often confer together. He was taking his first bite of scrambled eggs when I asked him, "Dan, do you know anything about AIDS?"

He shook his head, chewed and swallowed the bite. "Not much. Why? Got a patient?"

I nodded at him over my coffee cup. "Yes. My first one. An old Viet Nam buddy. A doctor. We operated together in Saigon. He dropped in yesterday afternoon. Surprised me. He looks awful."

"How do you know it's AIDS?"

"I don't. At least not for sure. He just came down from San Francisco. They diagnosed him up there. Couldn't do anything for him. So he came to me."

Dan raised his eyebrows. "Why's that?"

I shook my head. "He said nobody else can help him. And he thinks I can. Actually, he says I'm his last resort . . ." I set the cup down and twisted it slowly in my saucer.

"What're you going to do?" Dan asked slowly.

"I don't know. I just don't know. He brought me a copy of the workups the other doctors did. Haven't looked at them yet."

"Talked to anybody else about it?"

"No. You're the first one." I took a deep breath. "But I've got to do something, Dan. The guy's desperate. And scared."

Dan asked the inevitable. "Do you know if he's homosexual?"

"If there's anything I'm sure of, Dan, the guy's *not* homosexual!" Even as the words left my mouth I realized they sounded defensive. And in my heart I realized that was the question I'd been asking myself.

Dan raised his hands placatingly. "Okay, Bob. It's a natural question. One that everybody will ask . . ."

16

"I know, Dan. Sorry I spoke like that. But I *know* this guy." I thought a moment. "Well . . . at least I knew him. But it's been years since I saw him . . ."

Dan's question plagued me all morning.

Mary wasn't there when I drove home at noon. But she had prepared me a lunch. I carried it into my office and munched on it while I opened and read the contents of Roger Cochran's manila envelope. Twenty minutes later when I finished the last page, I suddenly realized most of my sandwich was still on the plate, uneaten. By that time I wasn't hungry any longer.

The reports raised more questions than they answered. All at once I realized that, other than the routine temp/pulse/respiration I had not examined Roger. I picked up my telephone and dialed my office. "Janine, see if you can get Roger Cochran to come in this afternoon."

It was nearly time to close the office before Janine ushered Roger into my examination room. Today I noticed that his feet seemed to hurt him, a fact I hadn't noticed yesterday. Besides looking more exhausted than before, if that were possible, Roger now looked apprehensive. He said nothing, but took his seat, looked at me expectantly and waited for me to speak.

I tapped his manila envelope. "I've gone over that," I said, "thoroughly . . ."

He nodded and crossed his legs to get more comfortable. When I didn't speak he asked, "Well, Bob, how does it look? Very bad? Or just medium bad?" He tried to chuckle at his attempted humor, but it came out as a raspy cough.

"Frankly, Roger, I'm not sure yet. I had a date last

night —with my wife. Anniversary. So I haven't had time to go over all the literature yet. There's a stack of it. But I've got to ask you some questions . . ."

"Shoot," was his simple response. His unblinking eyes never left my face.

". . . and examine you," I finished.

He arose. "The usual? Strip down to my skivvies?"

"Yes . . . I want to look at your feet and legs. The reports said something about some lesions."

Roger shrugged and began to unbutton his shirt.

I took a deep breath. "Roger, first a question . . ."

He looked at me. "Go ahead, Bob. Ask. Anything."

"The material I've been reading on AIDS . . ." I began, "all of it seems to indicate that . . ."

Roger interrupted me. ". . . that 80 to 90 percent of the victims are homosexual," he said with a tinge of sarcasm. "Is that what you want to know?"

I nodded mutely, embarrassed at his transparency.

He grinned for the first time today. "I thought you knew me better than that, Bob. Don't you remember those times in Saigon? And Sacramento?" He shook his head. "No, Bob. You can clear your mind of that possibility." He bent down and unlaced his shoes.

"Sorry, Roger. But you knew I'd have to ask . . ."

He looked up and grinned again. "Might interest you to know that for the last year or so I've been impotent. No activity of that kind at all. I've just been too . . . too weak." He stood to remove his trousers.

The emaciated physique Roger presented was a far cry from the perfect specimen I had seen in Viet Nam. He was panting heavily when he sat down and I could see his pulse throbbing in several places. Suddenly I resented the fact that he had come and had made me responsible for him. I didn't know this man anymore. But for some reason I couldn't be totally objective.

I sat on my stool and rolled over to him. I examined his arms, his neck, torso, legs, taking several minutes to run my fingers over his sagging skin, touching swollen lymph glands, checking muscle tone. Then, dreading to do so, I picked up one foot and saw what I had feared. He winced as I pressed gently on the dark red, raised lesion on the bottom of his foot.

"How long have you had that?" I asked.

He shrugged. "A month. Maybe longer."

"Know what it is?" I asked.

"No. Never saw one on anybody but myself . . . what is it? Jungle rot? Something I might have picked up in Viet Nam?"

I didn't answer, but picked up the other foot. It was worse than the first. A single vascular tumor covered nearly the entire soft part of his foot and two smaller ones were beginning to form along the calf of his leg. I touched them gently and felt him stiffen.

"Tender?" I asked.

"Very. What are they?"

I shook my head and answered slowly. "Roger, to be honest with you, I'm not sure . . ."

"But you think you know?"

I nodded.

He drew a deep, raspy breath. "Okay, Bob, level with me. What do you *think* it is?"

Before I answered, I turned and reached for my *Merck Manual, Fourteenth Edition*, scanned the index and turned to page 2077. I could almost feel Roger's eyes burning into my bent head. I ran my finger down the page, read it quickly, then turned the page.

"Find it?" Roger asked tonelessly.

"I think so," I said and handed him the open book.

Roger read both pages slowly, carefully and handed the *Manual* back to me. His face was ashen. "Kaposi's sarcoma! Good God, Bob. And you think *that's* what I've got?"

"Yes," I said, barely whispering the word. "I've got to do some more checking . . . but that's what it looks like."

CHAPTER FOUR

The examination finished for the moment, Roger
shuffled away and I sat disconsolately in the empty
examining room. It seemed like a huge dark cloud
had settled over me and I was having difficulty thinking. Vaguely I realized that Kaposi's saracoma was
one of those rare, exotic diseases that we'd touched
on in med school, but which, we were told, we would
probably never encounter in practice. So with the
mass of assigned "relevant material" with which we
had to familiarize ourselves, most of us, including
myself, gave KS hardly more than a cursory reading.

Now, it came to me with full force: Roger's life
might very well depend upon my gaining a quick and
intimate knowledge of the etiology and treatment of
those horrible-looking red blotches on his feet and
legs.

"Oh, God," I groaned, "where to begin?"

Fortunately, there was by 1985, a considerable
amount of material available on the subject. After I'd
seen my last patient for the day, I culled a huge arm-
load of pertinent journals from the growing stack
(with which I never quite got caught up), and carried
them home with me. Mary raised her eyebrows and

gave me a knowing smile when she saw me lugging them through the house. She knew what a doctor did with all those magazines.

I cleared my throat and began, "Hon, after dinner . . ."

"I know, Bob," she said, "you're going to your office and don't wish to be disturbed. Right?"

"You don't mind?"

She hugged me, journals and all. "Of course not. Do you think you're on to something?"

"I'm not sure," I said, "but maybe, just *maybe*, the secret of prolonging Roger's life might be hiding within these pages."

I scarcely tasted the meal Mary had prepared, though by the way the children devoured it, I'm sure it must have been a good one. They usually are. By seven-fifteen I was in my office, which I didn't leave until nearly ten o'clock, when I joined Mary in the family room for our nightly ritual: watching the evening news and getting caught up with the day.

Mary scooted close to me on the divan. "How's the research?"

"Okay," I said, nodding absentmindedly, because the first item on the news was a story about AIDS. At the commercial I clicked off the sound. "Nothing really new there," I said. "But I've learned something tonight that frightens me . . ."

"Something about AIDS?"

"Yes . . . and something to do with Roger's symptoms."

"Oh," she said, sitting up straight. "Want to talk about it?" When I nodded affirmatively, she took the remote from my hand and switched off the television.

For an hour or so I shared with her some of my findings. Kaposi's sarcoma, along with Pneumocystis pneumonia, I told her, are being associated with the diagnosis of AIDS more and more frequently.

"Where did AIDS come from?" she asked me. "Until a few years ago I don't remember ever hearing about it. Did you?"

I shook my head. "No, Honey, and that's really a strange thing. I'll get back to that in a minute. But first let me tell you what I've learned about KS—that's Kaposi's sarcoma. KS was first reported in Austria by a man named Kaposi. Moriz Kaposi. Between 1868 and 1871, Kaposi noted peculiar nodules or tumors 'brown-red to blue-red' in color about the size of 'peas or hazel nuts' on several patients who came to his dermatology clinic in Vienna. Kaposi observed that those tumors appeared first on the sole of the foot and the instep . . ."

I stopped talking abruptly and gazed at the now blank TV screen. Mary touched my arm and spoke softly. "And . . .?"

I cleared my throat. "Kaposi noted that those strange little tumors spread rapidly . . . and that they were usually lethal *within two to three years.*"

I took a deep breath. "Honey, it was tumors like Kaposi described that I found on Roger today."

"On his feet?"

"And his legs . . ."

She knew me well enough to know when I was upset, so she sat quietly beside me, gently massaging my neck and shoulders. After a few moments of silence, she asked softly, "Bob, what exactly are these tumors? Did you call them 'Kaposi's tumors'?"

"Yes. Kaposi's sarcoma. Nobody knows for sure what causes KS. Worse yet, nobody knows of any cure."

Mary is a good listener, and it helped me to verbalize some of the facts I'd been reading. Until recently, I told her, KS had been a very rare disease, and most physicians had never seen a case. Now that's all changed, I told her, "And in the past few years, the aggressive form of KS in association with AIDS has suddenly assumed epidemic proportions . . ."

Mary gasped, "In the USA?"

"And at least nine other countries."

"And you still don't know what causes this KS, *or* AIDS?"

I shook my head. "No. Not really. There are some educated guesses being made. But no real answers. No hard answers."

We sat in silence for a while. Mary sighed. "Bob . . . I, I still believe you'll do something for Roger. I really do."

"I hope so, Mary. I hope so."

Neither of us dropped off to sleep quickly. My mind was in a whirl. Lying in the darkness side by side, I said something I hadn't said for a long time. "Mary, the last few days I've found myself praying, you know? I haven't prayed much since 'Nam. But I want to help Roger. I've *got to* help Roger."

Mary's sleepy voice said, "Bob, I pray for you every day. Now I'll pray even more. G'night." She snuggled close to me and within seconds was breathing regularly.

"It just doesn't make sense!" I told David Cohen the next morning at the hospital. David and I had met at a convention in Seattle half a dozen years ago where he was visiting his parents. He had just completed interning at Bellvue in New York and was, as he put it, "Just shopping around . . ."

We struck up a friendship, and by the end of the week I invited him to join me in my growing practice. David agreed to "look it over," which he did a month later. Our wives liked each other immediately so David bought in. It had proven to be an excellent partnership.

"What doesn't make sense?" he asked me now.

"Kaposi's sarcoma. It's practically a death sentence. But its cause is unknown."

"Unknown?" he grimaced with a slight shrug. "But can't you say that about most diseases?"

"I guess you're right."

Most of my spare time the next weeks was spent researching AIDS. What I learned was more disturbing than enlightening. It was a rare newspaper or magazine or newscast that didn't carry at least one story about AIDS. Few conversations ended without a mention of the disease. Much that I heard was misinformation and conflicting. But of one thing I was certain: Our country, possibly our entire world, is gripped by AIDS hysteria.

Up till this point I had done nothing for Roger. I didn't know what to do. And each time I saw him I thought I noted a slight deterioration in his condition. Each time he shuffled away from me down the hall to go home it seemed that his shoulders slumped a little bit more.

One afternoon he looked especially bad. I tried to be brisk and cheerful, but my manner was phony even to myself. "I'm not doing so well am I, Bob?" he asked me.

"Holding your own isn't so bad," I said.

"Don't lie to me, Bob. We both know I'm not holding my own. Even I can tell I'm going downhill." He said it without rancor, almost without spirit. He rose and left without another word.

For the first time since I'd been practicing medicine, I was suddenly ready to chuck it all and go to sea.

From the time I learned to read at the age of five, I'd had two conflicting passions: to become a doctor and to become a sailor. For years I fluctuated between the two. First one, then the other was number one. By the time I was in high school I thought I might be able to combine the best of both worlds and become a seagoing doctor on a cruise ship.

My parents didn't know what to make of me. I specialized in two kinds of books at the library, and the librarians soon knew me, called me by name, and often held back new books from the racks for me to read.

I read every book the library carried on sailors, shipping and pirates. Pirates. I loved them and could quote their names, dates and conquests. I memorized the nomenclature of their ships, the number of guns they carried, and the seas they sailed. My best friend, Jonesy and I read those books together, reveled in the adventures of our heroes and planned further escapades of our own. We relived Tom Sawyer's short-lived pirating career, even to the point of building and launching a raft in the surf off Santa Monica Pier. This ill-fated cruise was rescued from ignominous extinction by the Coast Guard.

Happily for Jonesy and me, an amateur photographer recorded the event, which was properly heralded in the newspaper. Heroes for a day, we decided to quit while we were ahead and abandoned ships and shipping for the duration.

Shortly thereafter my medical preference took the ascendency and I began devouring *Gray's Anatomy* and books of its ilk. Soon my room became littered with anatomical reproductions of body organs and systems. I became obsessed with health and made everybody uncomfortable by diagnosing, prognosticating and even "curing" their ills. Admittedly my theories of longevity were influenced by my Sunday school theology, but I began questioning both my peers and elders concerning the present shortness of life as compared to Adam and his contemporaries.

"Why is our life span so short now?" I asked. "Those early Bible people lived hundreds of years and ours is only scores. Why? Did it have anything to do with their eating habits?"

The various—often contradictory—answers I received failed to satisfy, so I began researching my own questions. With my parents' permission (albeit their raised eyebrows) I purchased laboratory mice and set out to prove my theories. My lab soon overflowed my bedroom into the garage. I meticulously noted every detail concerning my mice, recording amounts and kinds of foods and fluids, number and sex of progeny, and—most importantly—apparent health and longevity.

I loved my mice and called them all by name. When I bought them from the laboratory supply through my high school science teacher, I asked, "How long do they live?"

"A couple of years. Maybe three. But that's only if you take good care of them."

I took good care of them, probably treated them better than I treated myself. They were my first and last thought of the day. I was especially fond of Adam and Eve—they were my first, and the parents of several generations of progeny.

My mice were separated into two control groups, and I was very careful to weigh and measure everything they ate. I soon noticed that the amount and kinds of food my mice ate made a huge difference in their vitality, their reproduction, as well as their longevity. By the time I graduated from high school and was ready for college, I had already developed some predictable curves for all three of these categories.

The Fall I entered UCLA was one of mixed blessings. I was ready, even eager, for college. But to maximize the experience I knew I should move into the dorm, which meant giving up my mice. So I stored my research and donated my mice, including Adam and Eve who, though ancient for mice (at that time they had reached the venerable age of 45 months!), were still living, to the high school science department. Before releasing them, I managed to elicit a sworn statement in blood that my mice would be cared for in the same manner to which they were accustomed, and that my record-keeping procedures would be continued.

Less than two months after they left my care and keeping, I was saddened to learn that Adam and Eve had both expired, within days of each other. Whether their deaths were due largely to old age or from a change of environment, I would never know. But I mourned their passing almost as I would the loss of human relatives and I moped about for days.

CHAPTER FIVE

I don't think David Cohen had ever seen me as angry as I was that afternoon as I stormed into the office looking, I'm sure, like I'd like to take somebody's head off.

"That guy thinks he's God!" I shouted.

"Who are you talking about?" he asked, apparently mystified.

"That radio preacher," I said. "Just happened to turn to his program on the way back from lunch. He said AIDS is a divine visitation of God . . . and that it's going to kill off one third of the whole human race! Ridiculous!"

"Who was he?"

"I didn't get his name. Wish I had. I just might call the radio station and find out." I found myself pacing nervously, waving my arms. "He said AIDS is the worst plague the world has ever known, and that we'd better get ready for it . . ."

David shook his head. "I know, Bob, I know. I hear that all the time . . ."

"But the man's wrong. Wrong. Wrong! All that preacher's doing is helping to spread panic. The public is already afraid to shake hands with their neighbors."

Later I pulled out my research: So far over 40,000 cases of AIDS had been reported, a mere 5,000 cases a year. And the media was whipping the people into a frenzy with its daily—almost hourly—reports of the new AIDS' inroads. I say a *mere* 5,000, because I knew that arteriosclerotic heart disease was claiming over 625,000 victims *annually*; that yearly cancer fatalities were approaching the half million mark; that more than a third of a million each year were succumbing to strokes; and that even osteoporosis deaths exceeded 300,000 annually.

Yet none of these killers had yet been labeled epidemic!

What's going on? I wondered. It almost seemed that there was an insidious scheme behind this proliferation of data concerning AIDS. I looked again at the reported facts: 70–90% of AIDS victims were known male homosexuals. Added to this list were the intravenous drug users, Haitian refugees, hemophiliacs, infants receiving blood transfusions, female sexual partners of males with AIDS, male prison inmates, female prostitutes.

In addition, the reports went, there were increasing numbers of victims that did not fit the above list. How did they fit in? There had to be a tie of some kind.

I went over the list again, asking myself, what did they all have in common? What was the essential ingredient of AIDS? The researchers said it was a virus. Perhaps it was. Perhaps not. One thing was certain, there *had to be a common link*, a universal common denominator. Somehow I could not believe that the "AIDS monster" was lurking behind every tree and stump, beneath every rock and in every alley, ready to pounce upon the unwary.

Despite the millions of dollars being spent upon research, no satisfactory answers to the conundrums surrounding AIDS have been found: Precisely what is AIDS? What is the cause? How is it transmitted? How can it be prevented? Can AIDS be cured?

Weeks into my research, I still had no clear idea as to the nature of AIDS. Even the symptoms for the disease were too vague and general, which could give rise to questionable diagnosis. I had listed them on a yellow pad. I reviewed them.

The most common signs and symptoms that suggest a *possible* diagnosis of AIDS are: swollen lymph glands for a period of time (I chuckled grimly. Even my own lymph glands were likely to swell at the most inopportune times for no apparent reason.), fatigue (What does that mean? All of us get tired, some of us more tired or more frequently tired than others. Witness the unending stream of tired-for-no-reason housewives that flows through my office.), fevers and night sweats (What did this mean? Many PMS patients regale me with these complaints.), weight loss (A relative "symptom" if it could be called a symptom.), diarrhea (Whenever I read a paper to my physician colleagues, or address the Optomists Club, I invariably get diarrhea; and my wife always does when my relatives come for an unannounced week-long visit).

I realized my list meant little, if anything. Because, in all the journals and reports I was reading it was reported that even though some or all of these symptoms *may be present* (though not necessarily) in homosexual or bisexual men (and other AIDS victims), in most instances Kaposi's sarcoma and/or other op-

31

portunistic infections such as Pneumocystis carinii do not develop.

With growing apprehension I realized that there was presently *no reliable method* for diagnosing AIDS. Worse than that, cancer patients receiving chemotherapy, and patients with hepatitis, infectious mononucleosis, and certain other diseases *may show immunosuppression similar to AIDS patients.*

This meant, and I shuddered as the thought came, that the diagnosis of AIDS by any physician would, of necessity, have to be largely *subjective.* That is, based on the measure of his or her diagnostic skills, and/or familiarity with the available material, the same patient seen by several physicians may or may not be diagnosed in the same manner.

"Dear God!" I burst out to Mary one evening in the family room after the children were in bed, "in the light of today's AIDS-panic-syndrome, a diagnosis of AIDS could very well become a death sentence."

Her face drained of color. "What do you mean?"

"The public is in such a panic that a person unfortunate enough to be diagnosed as having AIDS can be deprived of all his constitutional rights. All of them."

"Bob, but that's impossible."

"No, Mary, it is possible. And we're seeing it all around us." I ticked them off on my fingers. "Children being refused school attendance. County authorities removing children from AIDS-diagnosed parents. Adults with AIDS discriminated against in the work place. AIDS victims refused admission to public events and public conveyances. Just the other day a taxi driver refused to let Roger Cochran ride in his cab. And there's more . . ."

"That's terrible, Bob! How can this be happening to us?"

"Panic, Mary. Pure and simple. Mob mentality that no amount of correct information can prevent."

All of these thoughts plagued me constantly. But, as far as Roger was concerned, they were side issues, purely academic. And, I had to face the truth, as far as the main issue was concerned—the cure of his illness—I had made absolutely no discernible progress. I was totally stymied.

I groaned in mental anguish when I made that admission to my wife. Her answer startled me. "Bob, I don't pretend to know anything about AIDS, except what you tell me. But . . ."

She hesitated.

"Go on," I said. "But what?"

"Well, I was in the bookstore this week and I ran across a book . . . it didn't say anything about AIDS . . . but, it just might be saying something . . . something important . . ." With that she handed me a paperback book.

Shocked, I blurted out the title, "*Confessions of a Medical Heretic!*" I looked at her questioningly. "I don't understand. Why did you choose this particular book?"

"I'm really not sure," she said. "The title grabbed me. But the disclaimer above the title intrigued me. Read it."

I read, "*Caution: Medicine As Practiced in America Today May Be Dangerous To Your Health.*" I looked up, still mystified. And somewhat angry. "The guy's obviously a quack, Mary. Nobody but a quack would make such a statement."

She shook her head. "Don't be too quick to judge,

Bob. Read what's printed on the back of the
book . . ."
I turned the book over and read:

"Twenty-five years as a practicing physician have
convinced Dr. Mendelsohn that: * Annual physical
examinations are a health risk. * Hospitals are
dangerous places for the sick. * Most operations
do little good and many do harm. * Medical test-
ing laboratories are scandalously inaccurate. *
Many drugs cause more problems than they cure. *
The X-ray machine is the most pervasive and most
dangerous tool in the doctor's office."

"Who is this guy, Mary? I've never heard of him?"
"Go ahead, read the rest."

"Dr. Mendelsohn is a medical heretic," I read. "He
is also the Chairman of the Medical Licensing Committee for the State of Illinois, Associate Professor
of Preventive Medicine and Community Health in
the School of Medicine of the University of Illinois
and the recipient of numerous awards for excellence
in medicine and medical instruction. . . ."

I sat down slowly. The book seemed to burn in my
hands.
"Is something wrong, Bob?" Mary asked.
"Yes . . . no. I don't know. It's just that . . . well, I
don't know what to say about this . . . this book."
"Will you read it, Bob?"
I shrugged. "Do you think it's worth my time?"
She nodded emphatically. "Yes. I read quite a bit of
it this afternoon . . . and . . . and I think it makes
good sense."

"You do?" I was incredulous. "You really do?"

"Yes, I do. And, Bob, if you are really seeking a way to help your friend, I think you ought to at least listen to what Dr. Mendelsohn is saying."

She arose and put her arms around me. "Bob, I love you dearly. And I believe in you. But sometimes I think you've forgotten some of the high purposes you had when I met you . . . when you were a struggling medical student . . ."

My chest felt tight. My wife's words pounded on my ears. I didn't know how to respond. She kissed me lightly and stepped back. "Bob, I'm going to bed. I don't know what else you planned to do this evening. But, please, for my sake, as well as your own, please read what Dr. Mendelsohn has to say. Goodnight, Bob."

And then she was gone. I heard her high heels tapping down the hallway and up the stairs. Finally I heard her say goodnight to the children, and a few moments later close our bedroom door. I felt very much alone.

For a long moment her words rang in my ears. ". . . you've forgotten some of the high purposes you had when I met you . . ."

I was filled with mixed emotions. What right did she have to judge me? She had no medical training. She really didn't know what she was talking about. She knew nothing about diagnosing or treating patients. And she didn't know how hard I worked to provide her with a good life.

Suddenly angry, I slammed the book across the room. Angry words rose in my throat, but I held them in. Almost immediately I was sorry and ashamed of myself. Just as quickly as the anger came it was gone. Mary was a good woman. A good wife and mother. It had taken courage for her to do what she had done.

I picked up the book and smoothed its pages.

I guess I *should* read it. I turned my desk light on high and opened to what the author called "Non Credo." There he explained his position on Modern Medicine. In short, he was against it. I couldn't lay the book down now. I *had to* find out just exactly why he was against it.

I flipped through the chapter with growing incredulity. How could a medical doctor be so outspoken and not be ousted from practice? Time and again I pounded my fist on the desk to vent my feelings against . . . against what? Or whom? I wasn't certain. By the time I had finished the man's "Non Credo" I was shaken to the core of my medical being. I hated what Dr. Mendelsohn was saying. But I was forced to admit the truth of much of what he was saying.

I knew that it took guts for a doctor to so firmly and boldly think for himself, and then to put it in print for the whole world to read. I granted him my grudging admiration and turned to the first chapter which he had titled, "Dangerous Diagnosis," which he began with:

> "I don't advise anyone who has no symptoms to go to the doctor for a physical examination. For people *with* symptoms, it's not such a good idea either. . . ."

From that opening statement I was hooked. Admittedly I was intrigued, to say the least. Irritated, yes. Amused? Perhaps. But bored? Not a whit. How could I be when he wrote, "You should approach the diagnostic procedure with suspicion rather than confidence. . . ."?

What was Mendelsohn trying to do? Undermine the whole practice of medicine?

"You should be aware of the dangers," I read on, "and that even the simplest, seemingly innocuous elements can be a threat to your health or well-being. . . ."

Statements like this from an outsider could be ignored. But for *one of us* to be saying this truly was heresy. From such a beginning, wild horses could not have prevented me from reading the whole book. Mary was right, sane or not, this man just might have something of value to say.

Forgetting the time, I settled myself comfortably in my chair, adjusted the light again, and prepared myself for what could possibly become a rather enlightening hour or two with Dr. Robert S. Mendelsohn, self-acknowledged medical heretic.

CHAPTER SIX

Again and again as I read Mendelsohn's book, Roger Cochran came to mind. Especially when I came to the chapter, "Dangerous Diagnosis." "Doctors in general," he wrote, "should be treated with about the same degree of trust as used car salesmen. . . ."

That raised my hackles. But as I read on, I thought of Roger again. Could he trust me any more than he could trust a used car salesman? Perhaps one reason Roger was so concerned about his condition was because he did know so much. And because he knew that I knew so little about AIDS.

Dr. Mendelsohn's chapter on drugs disturbed me. Deeply. For months, perhaps years, I'd been concerned about the tremendous proliferation of drugs with which the pharmaceutical companies have been besieging the medical profession. It was getting so I hated to see that little man parked in my waiting room with his huge case of "samples" and "new drugs" to "combat" every disease listed in my *Merck Manual*.

But what could I do? I reasoned. I have to "keep up" with all the new stuff that's going on, don't I?

It was very late when I finished reading the book.

Though Mendelsohn hadn't won me over completely, I got his point.

I am not entirely sure why, but I didn't tell anybody at the hospital the next morning, not even my partner, Dr. David Cohen, about having read Dr. Mendelsohn's "Confessions . . ." Perhaps I was a little ashamed to have read something so derogatory to my chosen profession. Perhaps I was fearful that some osmotic process might also brand me as an heretic.

Nevertheless, I spoke of the book to no one. That is, to no one except Mary. As usual I had started my morning routine early without awakening her. But when I came home for lunch she met me with a warm hug and kiss. "Still angry, Bob?"

"I never was angry."

She laughed that special throaty laugh of hers that first attracted me to her. "Maybe not angry. But a little perturbed?"

I nodded. "A little. Just a little."

Her lunch was superb. While we ate, we spoke casually of the children and other non-threatening subjects, both of us studiously avoiding mention of *the book*. When we finished, she took my hand and led me into the family room. "Now, Doctor Bob, tell me what you thought of Dr. Mendelsohn's book."

I leaned back in my lounger. "Well . . ." I began, "what do you want to know first?"

"Did you like the book . . .?"

"No. Definitely not!" I broke in. "It's a disturbing book. Maybe even dangerous. A travesty . . ."

She smiled, untouched by my anger. "Then, Bob, why did you read it?"

I took the bait. "Because . . . because, Mary, because you wanted me to."

Her tinkle-bell laugh rang across the room. "And that was the *only* reason?"

Despite myself, I grinned. "Mary, you've done it again. You led me on, didn't you?"

She nodded.

"And you don't *really* care whether everything Mendelsohn is saying is true or not, do you?"

She shook her head. "No, Bob, I really don't. But I do care that you keep your mind alert. That you know what's being written by and about the medical profession. I want you to keep thinking—to think for yourself . . ."

"And to speak out, like Mendelsohn?"

"If need be, yes." She traced a pattern on the carpet with the toe of her sandal. "As you read the book, Bob, did something in it cause you to think of Roger?"

"Yes, several things."

"Such as?"

"The chapter on diagnosis. That disturbed me. The chapter dealing with drugs bothered me. A great deal. Drugging patients in an attempt to cure them bothers me. I've told you that before, haven't I?"

She nodded. "Yes, I thought of that, too."

"His chapter on preventive medicine also made me think of Roger. And I asked myself again, what does Roger *really* have? If he has AIDS, which he most likely does, what is AIDS? I've voiced these concerns to you a number of times during these past weeks."

"What are you going to do now?"

"About what?"

"Your concerns? About Roger? About everything in general?"

I took a deep breath. "You certainly know how to get me thinking again, don't you?"

"I hope so."

"Well . . . let's start with Roger. I'm going to get him in the office again—haven't seen him for a week or two—and get him talking. Get his opinion about this AIDS thing. In general *and* in relation to himself. I've got to admit I honestly thought he might have been lying to me about whether he was homosexual or not . . ."

"And you're not now?"

"No. Not really. Even though a very high majority of AIDS cases have been traced to homosexuality and its side effects. But Roger . . . Roger is different somehow. Mary, I know—I knew—Roger. I've seen him under fire, under pressure. I've been with him in social situation. I know how he responds to women. And women to him. I cannot believe Roger has any more homosexual tendencies than most men, myself included."

I checked my watch. "I've got to go in a couple of minutes. But, Mary, there is something in Roger's history that's been overlooked. By myself. By the other doctors. And that *something* is the key to his diagnosis. Perhaps to the diagnosis of all AIDS victims . . ." I rose to go.

Mary hugged me. "Bob, that's what I was hoping to hear."

"What's that?"

"Your own words, telling me that you're thinking, really thinking again. Don't trust anyone else's diagnosis, Bob. Don't even trust your own. I don't know all that's involved in diagnosing a patient, Bob, but I do know this—you are one of the most sensitive doctors I know. One of the most caring.

"But, more than that, you have a most unusual ability to touch, to feel, to think. And something even more important . . . to *sense* something unarticulated. And then to put it all together in a way that most doctors will never be able to do. And to come up with the answer that has completely baffled others. Even doctors with more experience than you . . ."

The glow of Mary's confidence followed me that afternoon. And I recognized something I hadn't realized: I had allowed myself to get into sort of a diagnostic rut. I had treated the "same old things" so much that I had allowed myself to become a little jaded, even bored with it all. I had become the sort of doctor they had warned me about in med school: The Doctor (with a capital "D") whom the patients regarded as God *until the doctor himself begins to believe and act as though he actually were God.*

"God help me," I thought. "I can't let that happen."

Three days later I arranged for Roger to come in. On purpose, I had scheduled him at three o'clock, the very last patient of the day. I hoped to enlist Roger's cooperation to help locate the missing link, that evanescent something, the universal, common denominator that *must be* present in all AIDS patients. Without that link I knew, we would forever treat symptoms instead of causes and administer Bandaids instead of eradicating disease.

Roger was five minutes early and looked like death warmed over. He greeted me with, "What's up, Bob?"

"Nothing new," I told him. "And that concerns me. I'm going to level with you, Roger." I indicated a stack of books and journals on my desk. "I've gone through all of this material. And I've come up with practically nothing."

He raised his eyebrows. "Nothing?"

"Not really nothing, Roger. Mostly conflicting

things. The medical records you brought with you show that your serum antibody tests indicate high levels of HTLV-III/LAV." I looked up. "You understand that, don't you?"

He nodded wearily. "Of course. In doctor jargon that's *human T-cell lymphotropic virus Type III lymphadenopathy-associated virus*. But, it sounds like some sort of double talk to me. What does it mean to you?"

"To be honest, Roger, I don't know. I think it's anybody's guess. We could probably go all around the barn philosophizing the medical implications of that definition, but in the end we'd be right back on square one."

Roger's shoulders sagged. "Then we're actually nowhere, Bob. Is that what you're telling me?"

"Yes and no. I think by now you know that I've done a lot of reading—and thinking—about this whole AIDS thing these past few weeks. I've learned a lot. Probably not much more than you've learned about AIDS. I now know the highest at risk groups. You know them as well as I . . ."

"Then what are you getting at?"

"I think I'm getting warm. I'm not positive, but I think so. Now I've got to know more than I know. A whole lot more. And you've got to help me.

"There are some missing pieces to the puzzle, Roger. And so far none of the researchers seem to have found them." He started to speak but I held my hand up.

"Let me finish this thought. So far, Roger, it seems that most of the researchers' focus is on the sex transmissibility of AIDS. At this point I can't prove or disprove the truth of that thesis . . ."

Roger broke in angrily. "Bob, I've already told you that I'm straight! Don't you believe me, man?"

"Hold it, Roger. You're jumping the gun. I *do believe you.* And that's just the point. I've got a gut feeling that something else is responsible. Something more universal than sex that's responsible for this so-called epidemic we're calling AIDS."

"What's more universal than sex?" Roger asked drily.

"Don't get cynical on me, Roger. Just listen. *Listen.*"

"Okay, I'm listening."

"Don't listen like a patient. Listen like a doctor. Better yet, listen like *both* a doctor and a patient. Which is literally what you are. Can you do that?"

"I'll try."

"Okay, Roger, I've got to ask you some straight questions. And I've got to have honest answers. Strictly honest. No holds barred. Okay?"

Roger tensed perceptibly. "Okay, okay. Ask."

"You were on hard drugs in Viet Nam. Right?"

"Sure, Bob, you knew I was!"

I nodded. "Did you ever kick the needle. I mean, totally?"

"What are you getting at?"

"Just answer the question. Did you ever get off the needle? Completely off the needle?"

"Yes, I did. It took me a while, but I did."

"Tell me about it, Roger. This is *very important*—not just to your case, but to research as a whole."

"For a while after 'Nam I was still shooting up. I had to, Bob. I was sick. I don't think I ever got over 'Nam. But I was an outpatient at the Veteran's Hospital for years. They got me off the needle. But I still took drugs. Prescription drugs."

Roger looked miserable. I knew I was getting somewhere. I couldn't let up. I had to go on. "I want to be sure that my facts are accurate. Even though you were in private practice in San Francisco, as an outpatient of the Veteran's Hospital, you were still taking drugs?"

"Yes, that's right."

"Another question: Roger, were you ever discharged from the Veteran's Hospital in San Francisco?"

"No. Never was."

"And all the time you were an outpatient you were taking drugs. On legitimate prescriptions?"

"I don't know what you're getting at. But, the answer's yes."

I checked Roger's records. "You practiced down in the Haight area of San Francisco, didn't you?"

Roger just nodded.

"Many of your patients were gay, weren't they?"

Another nod.

"Did any of them have AIDS?"

"Yes. Several of them." Roger sat up straight. "Do you think I caught AIDS from treating them?"

I shook my head slowly. "No, Roger, I don't think so. I don't think that's possible. Apparently the AMA agrees with me. So does *The New England Journal of Medicine*." I indicated an article in my February 6, 1987 issue. "You can read it later if you'd care to . . ."

"I'll take your word for it," Roger said. "But what I want to know is: What exactly are you getting at?"

"Just a few more questions, and I'll tell you what I think." I referred again to his medical history. "About a year ago you entered the Veteran's Hospital with symptoms similar to those you have now. Right?"

"Right. At first they thought I had pneumonia . . ."

"Then they discovered a tumor in your abdomen?"

Roger nodded.

"And you were given radiation therapy, followed by chemotherapy? After which you have never fully regained either your full weight or your strength? Is that right?"

"Exactly right. Now will you tell me . . ."

"In just a minute. In an attempt to regain your lost weight you began forcing yourself to eat heavily. Including lots of rare steaks and sushi."

"How did you know all this," Roger asked. "It's not all in my medical history."

I shrugged. "Elementary. I just talked to your doctor at the Veteran's Hospital. He told me. Anyway, you began gaining weight—though you didn't regain what you had lost. But you noticed that your blood pressure rose alarmingly . . ." Another nod. "So you began taking diuretics, as prescribed by your doctor?"

"Right on all counts," Roger said. "You should have been a medical detective."

"Isn't that what a good doctor is?" I asked. Before he could respond I said, "That's about when the headaches began, isn't it? And you began to lose the weight you'd gained? And then came the fatigue . . . the terrible exhaustion . . .?"

My patient nodded. "And speaking of exhaustion, Bob. Can we finish this another time? I've just got to get to bed . . ."

I looked at my watch. We'd been at this for nearly two hours. "Okay, Roger. I'll take you home . . ."

In the car I asked, "What are you having to eat tonight?"

Slumped beside me, Roger barely mumbled. "Don't know. Don't have much in my room. Don't feel like going out to eat."

I stopped at a supermarket and loaded up on some things for him. And when we got to his hotel, I carried a couple of bags of food to his room. He seemed to revive a trifle when he got to his door.

"Just set the stuff on the floor there," he said. "I appreciate all you're doing. Now, can you tell me in a word what it is you think you're on to?"

"Yes, Roger. It's just this . . ." Speaking rather fast, in a few terse sentences I outlined my preliminary conclusions. When I finished, Roger gave me a weak, though wan smile. "Then you think there's still a chance? Still time . . . for me?"

I pulled his emaciated body to me. "I think so, buddy. I hope so . . . I really do."

"Thank God," he said and inserted his key in the door.

CHAPTER SEVEN

Med school was tough going, all the way through. In fact, in my rather sheltered life, I'd never encountered anything that could hold a candle to it. The closest thing that came to it was the summer I had crewed on a sailing race to Hawaii. The captain took the race seriously and I worked—all of us did—harder than I had ever worked in my life. From early morning till late we trimmed sail, put on sail, put out the balloon jib, trimmed the boat, till I thought I'd go out of my mind.

Then we'd grab a bite to eat and a couple hours sleep and go at it again. I'd never though a "cruise" would turn out like that. In the end we won the race, but by that time I was so tired that I hadn't cared.

Med school was sort of like that. In a way. It was tough and demanding. But interning was worse. There were days when I didn't think all this was worth it. Those 24-hour plus duties were killers. I hated them, as did all the interns. Fortunately (or unfortunately, depending upon your point of view), for me and a few others, Viet Nam came along. At least that's what I thought at first.

But it wasn't. It was hell. I've spent these last years just trying to forget the horrors of that hell. Sometimes I wake up screaming, reliving . . . amputating shredded limbs. Trying to piece together land mine victims. Seeing, hearing the shelling of our hospital, the horror of patients trapped beneath burning debris . . .

Even Dante couldn't have painted hell any more realistically.

I learned a lot though. I learned how to work under pressure—how to ignore fatigue and hunger. To work like an automaton. The sweet taste of success and victory when a patient lived. The acid taste of failure when Charley won and the patient died. I learned the worth of the precious gift of life . . .

It's kinda funny, I thought, those months in Viet Nam taught me more than all the books and lectures and demonstrations. All of that was necessary, but when I came out of med school I was a raw, green kid. Cocky. Jaunty. And all that. But I didn't know anything about medicine. Or surgery.

I found that out when I got my first experience in Surgery. I was ready, oh, how I was ready. I thought. It was to be an appendectomy. Simple and basic. Hadn't I seen a dozen or more of them? Along with a bunch of other procedures? Of course. I'd read all the texts, heard all the lectures, watched the masters at work. Nothing to it.

I brushed up on the section on appendectomy in my treasured *Atlas of Operative Technique*. The hour came and I meticulously prepped the patient and scrubbed up. Then, gowned, gloved and masked, I took my place on the right side of the operating table. The veteran surgeon who was "assisting" me nodded. I motioned to the nurse and she slapped the scalpel in my hand. I traced an imaginary line on the draped abdomen, and . . .

And froze.

All my confidence and cocksureness fled. My mind went blank. Sweat poured down my back. I gripped the scalpel and leaned over the patient. Suddenly I was aware of the patient. It wasn't a cadaver. It was a real, live human being. And I was about to have the temerity to cut him open.

With the help of my "assistant" I finally managed to do the right things. Two hours later (I should have done it in one) I closed, thanked the nurse and anesthesiologist. Nodded my gratitude to my assistant. And fled.

The patient recovered and was none the worse. I recovered as well. Gratefully . . .

Sitting alone now in my dark, empty office, I remembered that first attempt to achieve in actuality something I had already achieved intellectually and philosophically. There was a huge gulf fixed between the mind and the hand. Between the "knowing" and the accomplishing.

Roger Cochran's face fixed itself in my mind, where it had resided for weeks. I had promised to help him. Now I was face-to-face with the fact that I did not possess the knowledge to do it. What did I need? Research.

I had studied research. Like I had studied medicine. I had read the books, attended the lectures, admired the researchers. Mentally I understood research. Now I had to do it.

I looked at the stack of papers, journals and books before me. Roger's plain manilla envelope lay beside the stack. Perhaps some sort of symbolism, I thought. Within that stack of paper were all the pieces of the

puzzle. Now, all I had to do was to put them together. And make them fit.

Jigsaw puzzles. Not my thing. On rare occasions
I'd been trapped into starting one. I did alright with
the borders and some of the center (as long as the
pattern was in front of me, though I was lost without
it). But when it came to completing the puzzle, the
last score of pieces *would not fit*. I could have sworn
that some were missing.

Once when I had come down to the last pieces,
and finding none that would fill in those remaining
gaping holes, I had groaned in frustration and swept
the whole thing onto the floor.

But I couldn't do that now. The puzzle was AIDS.
The prize for completion was Roger's life. "Oh,
God . . . I don't know how to finish the puzzle. I
don't know how . . ."

Dr. David and I were seated in his favorite restaurant in West LA where we held our weekly partnership lunches. Over a kosher corned beef on rye, I
began. "David, I've never been so frustrated in my
life . . ."

He chewed and swallowed a bite. "Roger Cochran?"

"Yes. And AIDS."

"Know what you mean," he said. "I've got this little
boy, he's about three. All sorts of wierd symptoms.
Don't know quite what to make of them." He finished
off his sandwich and leaned back in his chair. "Okay,
Bob, let's get on with it."

"It's AIDS. And Roger Cochran. It's like I'm trying
to piece together a huge jigsaw puzzle. You know
how I hate those things. And I'm down to the last
few pieces. But they won't fit. So the puzzle is unfinished. The last pieces are missing. It's driving me

crazy. And time is running out for Cochran."

"What missing pieces are you looking for?"

"David, there's got to be a thread, a common denominator that runs through all the cases of AIDS. It isn't homosexuality. Because there are victims of AIDS who are straight. It isn't sex even. Because there are proven cases that are non-sex related. I don't know what it is, but there's a missing piece. And I don't know what it is."

David took a sip of water and nodded. "I agree. Any ideas?"

I shook my head. "Not yet. I've read about everything there is on the subject. All the journals, magazine articles, reports, books. You name them and I've either read them or know what they say."

"And . . ." David said, knowing there was more coming.

"And they all sound like Establishment propaganda."

David chuckled. "You mean the American Medical Association? Sounds heretical to me, Bob."

"Maybe so," I said. "But the AMA and the Center for Disease Control in Atlanta—they're both saying about the same things . . ."

"And what's that?"

"Like . . . well, both the AMA and the CDC are pouring out news releases for the media. Radio. TV. Newspapers . . . magazines. They keep feeding the world statistics—40,000 victims today, 50% of them dead. Inciting the public to panic. That sort of thing. They talk about: great progress being made, new vaccines and drugs . . ."

I stopped suddenly.

"What's the matter?" David asked. "Think of something?"

"I'm not sure, David. Not sure." I picked up the tab. "Let's go and I'll tell you about it on the way back to the office."

While David skillfully wove his way through the traffic, I told him, "I think I've got something. I think I have . . ."

"Got what?" David pulled up behind the office and turned off the engine. "You've got what, Bob?"

"I'm not sure . . . but I think I know what one of the missing pieces is."

"If you do, Bob, you've got a winner. And maybe even the Nobel Prize."

"Right now I'm not concerned about that. Listen . . ."

For the next ten minutes I shared with him what I believed to be at least *part* of the missing link of the disease that many researchers and certainly the news media call the plague of the century. David listened intently. And when I finished speaking, he spoke thoughtfully.

"Bob . . . I don't know. I've got to think about that. It, well, it sounds so, so simplistic . . ."

"And too obvious. I know, but I can't shake the thought."

He checked his watch. "We've got to get in there, Bob. But let me think about it. Okay? Then let's talk again."

I nodded. "Maybe tomorrow?"

"Yes. But, anyway, thanks for sharing your thoughts with me."

The rest of the afternoon went by in a haze. In my heart I knew I was right. But where was I to go from here? When I shared the idea with Mary, she was first excited, then became very sober.

"That covers the cause," she said. "But what about the cure? In other words . . ."

". . . what about Roger?" I finished for her, then added. "I don't know. But at least it's a beginning."

CHAPTER EIGHT

When I arrived at the office the next afternoon Roger was waiting for me. "I couldn't sleep all night," he said. "Your idea excited me so much that I just had to see you." He looked like he'd been up all night.

"When's my first appointment?" I asked Janine.

"One thirty," she said. "You've got about half an hour."

"Good," I said. "Roger and I will be in my office."

I closed the door and motioned Roger to a chair. I pulled one up close to his. "We don't have much time right now," I told him. "Let's get right to work. What do you have?"

Roger opened up a notebook. "Your *common denominator* idea is the most logical one I've heard yet. So I've been listing all the ones that seem to have common characteristics."

"How many do you have?"

"Several. I've listed even the most obvious," he began. "No special order, but the first one is: AIDS strikes both sexes, but not equally. More males than females. No clear reason for the apparent inequality."

I nodded. "Okay, I agree . . . let's move on."

"My next observation," Roger said, "is that one's age seems to have little to do with his or her susceptibility to AIDS." He looked up. "Of course, I realize that there *are* more adults than youth or children with AIDS. At this point that may or may not be an important distinction."

"I agree."

"Third observation: Life expectancy after diagnosis seems to be the same for male or female regardless of age." He checked his notes. "And that's approximately 35 to 40 months. Right so far?"

"Check."

"Sexual activity *seems* to be a predominant factor. By that I mean, there's a higher percentage of AIDS victims that are sexually active than those who are not."

"You're right on, Roger. Keep going. We've still got a little time left."

"Fourth observation: Without exception, at least that I could determine from the facts available, *every single person* diagnosed as having AIDS had been *traumatized* in some manner for a period of time— either physically, emotionally, sexually, chemically or, I guess you could say, medically."

"That's very good, Roger!" I said. "Very good. I think we're getting somewhere . . ." At that moment Janine tapped on my door. "Doctor Bob, your first patient is in Examining Room A."

"Thanks, I'll be right there." I stood up and gripped Roger's hand. The new light in his eye was heartening. "Sorry that I've got to leave you now. I'd like to go over the rest of your observations with you this afternoon. Can you wait?"

Roger grinned his lopsided grin. "Sure, Bob. I'm not going anywhere. May I wait in here?"

"Sure, take a look at my recent AMA journals . . .
or whatever. I'll pop in when I can."

The afternoon was very heavy and it was nearly
five before I got to talk to Roger again. I had looked
in a time or two, but he was asleep on the divan and
I didn't waken him. I was very eager to listen to his
other observations.

By the time I had finished with my last patient,
Roger was awake and writing in his notebook.

"Sorry," I said as I took off my white smock and
relaxed in my high-back desk chair. "It's been one of
those days."

Roger finished writing what he was working on
before he responded. "It's okay, Bob. Got a lot
done . . ."

"Like a long nap?" I teased.

"Sure, why not. I haven't slept in a doctor's lounge
since I interned. Felt good."

I looked at my watch. "Say, Roger, I've got an idea.
Why don't I call Mary. If nothing special's planned
for the evening maybe you could come home with
me . . ."

"Hold it, Bob," he said. "That's hardly fair to your
wife."

"Nonsense. She'd like to meet you. She's talked
about having you over. This might be a good time."

"But . . . isn't she afraid? Of AIDS . . . and the
kids?"

"Mary's not afraid of AIDS, Roger. She's kept right
up on my research with me. And the kids . . . well,
it'll do you good to talk to youngsters again." I
reached for the phone.

"Hi, Hon, Roger's in my office with me. And I
thought . . ."

I knew I could depend upon Mary. She beat me to

the punch and invited Roger. When I relayed her invitation, Roger was visibly moved. "I haven't been in a private home for a long time," he said. I was ashamed I hadn't invited him before.

And hour later Mary was serving us one of her well-planned dinners. Julie and Bobby were their usual vivacious selves and Roger was quickly at ease. About midway in the meal Julie surprised me, and all of us.

"Doctor Cochran, do you have AIDS?"

Mary's face went pale. "Why, Julie! Such a question."

I wasn't sure what to expect from Roger, but I shouldn't have been concerned. "Roger," I began, "I'm sorry . . ."

He grinned lopsidedly at me. "Bob, it's perfectly alright." He smiled at our 10-year-old daughter. "Yes, young lady, I have AIDS. What do you know about AIDS?"

She looked to Mary, then to me before answering. I nodded. "Go ahead, Julie."

"Well, Mother and Daddy didn't tell me. But I heard them talking about you one night. And, well, Mother said she would have you over for dinner one night. So, I . . ."

Roger laughed. It sounded good. I hadn't heard him laugh since he'd come to my office. "So you just put two and two together. Right?"

She nodded. "I guess so."

"Anyway, Julie," Roger said, "just what do you know about the disease I've got? About AIDS?"

I was amazed at what she told us. Julie is quite bright and is enrolled in a gifted child program. One of her teachers had talked to the class about AIDS. Quite unselfconsciously, Julie said, "Mrs. Joplin told us that a lot of people are getting AIDS. Then she explained what AIDS stands for . . ."

"And what does it stand for?" I asked.

"AIDS means acquired immune deficiency syndrome," Julie responded quickly. "It means that the immune system of the person who has AIDS isn't working properly. I guess that means that bad things made their immune system quit working."

Roger and I exchanged glances. "What kind of bad things do you think might do this?" I asked.

Julie shook her head. "I don't know. But I heard some teachers say that some people do bad things with sex. But I don't know what they meant." She shrugged. "Maybe the people who get AIDS misuse drugs . . . you know, use too many drugs. Or, maybe they use drugs in ways they aren't supposed to be used. I just don't know . . ."

Julie turned her innocent blue eyes upon Roger. "Doctor Cochran, do you misuse drugs? Maybe that's why your immune system quit working. Do you suppose?"

I was startled by Julie's "misuse drugs" question. Suddenly I was aware that I'd been holding my breath. I let it out slowly.

Roger had paused, a forkful of food on its way to his mouth. "Perhaps so, Julie," he said. "Perhaps so. Anyway, thank you for sharing your understanding of AIDS with us."

Under his breath, he added, so low that nobody but Mary and I heard, "Out of the mouths of babes . . ."

Mary was looking from one to another of the three of us. "What's going on? I seem to be missing something. Am I?"

"Hon, you're not missing anything. Nothing at all.

But it just *could be* that our daughter might have put her finger on another missing piece to the AIDS puzzle." I slid my chair back and went around the table to where my daughter was sitting with a questioning look on her face.

"What did I do, Daddy?"

I hugged her. "Julie, I think you might have helped your daddy to find a way to help people who've got that awful disease. Thanks. Thanks a lot. Right, Roger?"

Roger wasn't speaking. He was weeping unashamedly.

Later, in my office, I pulled out the familiar yellow lined tablet. "Roger, let's consider that drugged aspect. First, let's consider you. Would Julie's definition fit you in any way?"

He nodded. "Very definitely. To begin with, in 'Nam I was taking hard drugs. That's drug abuse. Then, back in the States I was still taking drugs . . ."

"Prescription drugs?"

"That's right. But hard drugs just the same."

"And you've actually been taking drugs—legitimate drugs, but drugs just the same—from then until now?"

"Sorry to say, Bob, but the answer's yes."

"Then you were hospitalized, with symptoms similar to the ones you have now. Right?"

He shook his head. "They thought I had pneumonia . . ."

"More drugs?"

"More drugs."

I was talking faster now. Things were beginning to add up. "Then the tumor in your abdomen . . . radiation therapy . . . and chemotherapy?"

"Yes, yes, yes. Yes to all of those."

"Then the high blood pressure. And more drugs? Some of which you're still taking to this very day?"

Roger nodded miserably. "Like Julie said, Bob. People did bad things to their bodies and their immune systems stopped working. Is that what you're getting at?"

I thought a minute. "Roger, I want this to come out right. It's been in my mind in sort of a jumbled form for several days. But tonight the pieces are getting sorted out . . . they're beginning to fit into the right places . . ."

I paused to put the words in order in my mind.

"I'm listening, old buddy," Roger said. "Shoot!"

"Roger, all along we've been told—and we've swallowed the concept—that AIDS *attacks* its victims. Right?"

"Right. That's been my understanding. Like I just happened to be in the wrong place at the wrong time and this evil spirit or demon got me."

"That's it. You might have had sex with the wrong partner . . . or the wrong kind of sex . . . or you shot up with a contaminated needle . . . or you're a hemophiliac and you receive a wrong batch of blood, or contaminated blood . . . or you're a babe in the womb and your mother was hooked on drugs and you got contaminated in the amniotic fluid . . ."

"Right, right!" Roger nearly shouted. "Or you had cancer or an organ transplant and were given immunosuppressive drugs . . ."

I paused, aware that my heart was pounding. "Roger, what's the common denominator in all of these things. Before you answer, it's *not* a virus, is it?"

He was shaking his head. "No, Bob. Not a virus

63

that gotcha. It was drugs. Drugs and more drugs."

"Or heavy abuse. Like homosexual abuse . . ."

Even as I said that, a light went on inside my head. "Roger, I've got it. I've got it!" I was pacing around like a caged tiger, unaware that Mary had entered the room and was standing quietly inside the door.

"Listen. AIDS is not a disease epidemic at all. *AIDS is an epidemic of abusive lifestyles*! Put another way: AIDS does not destroy the immune system. But a weakened immune system falls prey to a combination of symptoms that we call AIDS! Roger, AIDS doesn't *cause* a non-functioning immune system. AIDS is the *result* of an already non-functioning immune system!"

Suddenly Roger and Mary began applauding.

Mary ran and leaped into my arms. "Bob, I'm proud of you. For the first time AIDS makes sense to me. I believe you are right. Oh, I'm so proud of you. I love you, Bob!"

I hugged her back, lifted her from her feet and spun her around. "Mary . . . Roger, we don't have to be afraid of a virus we can't see. Never. But we do have to be aware of pushing our wonderful bodies past the breaking point . . ."

Roger spoke up. "That's a good definition, Bob. AIDS is an example of our bodies abused beyond the breaking point: that's AIDS!"

CHAPTER NINE

I *knew* I was right. It felt good. It sounded good. It *was* good. I somehow was certain of this fact: AIDS is the result of immune systems stretched to and beyond the breaking point. When the immune system can no longer cope, stretch no further, respond no more, it reacted like Longfellow's "Wonderful One Hoss Shay." In his immortal ballad, this shay was built of the best materials in the land and was designed to last 100 years and a day.

Which it did. Then, the moment the time for its demise was reached and exceeded, the wonderfully-built buggy fell apart *all at once*, and crumbled into dust. Though not exactly a parallel, when the immune system exceeds its limit (be it only one year or 100), it ceases to function and the body quite literally quickly "falls apart" and death results.

Something about the manner in which AIDS is said to "attack" its victims reminds me of the "Wolf, wolf!" fable I heard as a child, where a prankster repeatedly warned his shepherd friend that wolves were coming. Each time he heard the warning, the shepherd rallied his sheep and prepared to defend them.

Then the prankster laughed, "I fooled you! There aren't any wolves."

But he enjoyed his game so much that he tried it again and again, each time inciting alarm and subsequent preparedness by the shepherd. One day the shepherd tired of the game and ignored the warning. This time, however, the alarm was genuine. When the shepherd failed to respond, the prankster shouted, "The wolves are really coming this time. Please get ready!"

The shepherd laughed, "You have fooled me too many times. I won't fall for your game any more."

As a result, the shepherd refused to respond to the warning. He refused to rally and protect his sheep from the impending danger. And the wolves pounced upon the sheep and killed them.

When our immune systems get "fooled" again and again, they get tired, exhausted, wear out and cannot respond to the crises when they come. It is then that the body falls prey to what the researchers call "opportunistic diseases" such as Kaposi's sarcoma and Pneumocystis carinii. It is then that the victim is diagnosed as having the "dread, fatal disease" we recognize as *Acquired Immune Deficiency Syndrome* or AIDS.

Though I believed I was on the right track, as a scientist I realized I hadn't proven anything. I had developed a thesis, but now I had to prove it. This, I realized, could become a task far more difficult than anything I had yet accomplished.

Nevertheless, I had reached the watershed. In good conscience retreat was impossible. I could only advance.

Lying awake that night, I suffered pangs of self-doubt. At the moment of revelation, it had seemed almost too pat, too easy. Despite the weeks of searching, of wandering in the wilderness and maze of medical/pharmaceutical hype and doubletalk, I now wondered if my definitions of AIDS weren't too glib, too smooth.

But even if I was on the right track, what could I do? What better alternative could I offer? Could I refuse drugs and medications to my patients? Weren't some drugs helpful? Necessary? What about diuretics? Tranquilizers? Simple pain medications? Heart medications? Did they, too, fit the categories of abuse that Roger and I had defined?

Could our civilization function without drugs?

And, even if I could solve that problem, and could answer that question to the satisfaction of my colleagues and patients, what could I do about Roger? About all AIDS victims? Could I blithely condemn them for their "drug abusive" lifestyle and then leave them to their own devices to solve their terminal condition the best way they could?

Roger . . . Roger . . . Roger. What about Roger? When I dropped him off at his hotel he was elated. He, too, believed that we had located a missing piece. But, I asked myself again, *so what*? How would all this academic cerebration ultimately affect him?

Could our discovery halt his AIDS in its tracks? Could it stem the tide? Would it, could it save his life?

As the night hours ticked into eternity, I alternately scaled the Everest of the sublimity of victory, only to slip from my lofty perch to plumb Dante's depths of despair.

What can I do about Roger?

He and I had agreed to meet for lunch the following day to brainstorm and regroup. For the first time since he'd appeared in Los Angeles, Roger was in a jovial mood. "Order up, buddy," he commanded. "It's on me this time."

I started to protest, but he held up his hand. "Forget it. Remember, 'The condemned man ate a hearty dinner.'"

I made a face and he laughed. "Okay, okay. Let's put it this way, the *formerly* condemned man ate a hearty dinner. How's that?"

"Better," I admitted. "Okay, you're on . . ."

I ordered a salad and whole grain toast with just water to drink. Roger protested. "Is that all? Have you forgotten who's paying the tab."

"That's all I ever eat at lunch. Thanks just the same."

Roger ordered a small steak, well done, with fries and a large Coke. Before he tasted either the steak or the fries he liberally sprinkled them with salt. Neither of us said much while we ate. When we finished eating, I sipped my water and he ordered coffee, with cream, and spooned in several teaspoons of sugar.

He tasted his coffee and made a face. "Too strong." And added more sugar. He tasted it again. "Just right. I've been hooked on this stuff since med school. What about you?"

I shook my head. "I haven't touched coffee for years."

He shrugged. "Okay, Bob, let's go at it again. After you've had time to think about it a while, what do you think of your pet AIDS thesis? Personally, I think it's great. I went home last night and slept better than I've slept in months. I honestly believe there's help in sight . . ."

I sipped my water and merely nodded.

He set his cup down. "Don't you agree, Bob? You

do agree, don't you?" There was an edge of concern in his voice.

"Roger, I do believe I'm right. Or, we're right, because we're both in this together. But, even if we're on the right track—and I honestly believe that we are—we've got a very real problem to solve."

"What's that?"

"Roger, even if we ceased drugging our patients . . . and, believe me, that's a biggy with the Medical and Pharmaceutical Establishment, we've got another one just about as big. And that's the one that really concerns me."

Roger absentmindedly spooned more sugar into his coffee and stirred it. "I guess I don't understand. What do you mean?"

I drew a deep breath. "Roger, to put it bluntly, it's the matter of *reversing* the suppression of the immune system. If the immune system has ceased to function, or nearly so, what's going to get it going again?"

Roger visibly paled. "I guess I thought that all you had to do was just have the patient quit taking drugs . . . don't you?"

I shook my head. "No, Roger, I don't think it's quite that easy."

"But why not?" He drained his cup and accepted a refill from the waiter, loading it with cream and sugar as he had done before. "If drugs caused the problem in the first place, removing the drugs should reverse the problem. Right?"

"Yes and no."

He frowned. "That yes and no routine again. It's either yes or no. But not both. Give it to me straight."

I uncrossed my legs and leaned toward him. "Okay, Roger, you want it straight. I'll give it to you straight. This is your doctor speaking now. Okay?"

"Yes, sure. What's that supposed to mean?"

"Roger, how much coffee do you drink in a day? Five cups? Ten? More?"

"A dozen. Maybe fifteen. More or less."

"And half a dozen teaspoons of sugar in each one?"

"I guess. Never counted. What are you getting at?"

"Okay, Roger. Last night when I was talking about an abusive lifestyle, you thought I was talking about drugs, didn't you?"

"Yeah, I did. Hard drugs. Prescription drugs. Chemotherapy. That sort of thing. But coffee?"

"Yes, coffee. And tea. And chocolate. And Coke. They all contain caffeine. Lots of caffeine. Do you remember your freshman Chemistry. Caffeine is a drug . . ."

Roger burst out laughing. "Come off it, Bob. *Everybody* drinks coffee. And *everybody* drinks Coke. Are you trying to tell me that the two hundred million Americans who drink coffee are addicted to a drug? That's crazy!"

"That's precisely what I'm telling you, Roger. And if you don't believe me, just try to kick the habit. You'll suffer withdrawal *exactly* like you did when you kicked hard drugs."

Roger laughed again. "You've gotta be kidding? Anyway, what's that got to do with AIDS?"

I wasn't smiling when I responded. "Roger, remember, you're the patient and I'm the doctor. I'm going to take you back to 'Nam for a couple of minutes . . ."

"Okay, you're the doctor. I'll go along with you."

"Do you remember the GI's we operated on, the ones with gut wounds?"

"Sure, how could I forget."

"How old were those men. On the average?"

He looked puzzled. "I don't get it?"

"Go on, Roger, tell me. How old would they be. Would the average be twenty? Twenty-five? Thirty? Pick a number."

He shrugged. "Oh, twenty, twenty-two, I'd guess. Why?"

"Do you remember how many of those men had arteriosclerosis? Hardening of the arteries? And high blood pressure?"

"Yeah, sure. Most of them did. But I *still* don't know what you're getting at."

"And how about yourself? Don't you have high blood pressure? Don't you have trouble climbing stairs? Don't you . . .?"

Roger held up his hand. "Okay, okay, Bob. Get to the point. What's any of this got to do with AIDS? Or does it?"

"Roger, all of this has *everything* to do with AIDS. Your AIDS. Anybody's AIDS. When I was talking about an abusive lifestyle last night, I was referring to abuse of any kind. of *every* kind. Don't you get it, Roger? Abuse of the body includes drugs. But it also includes overindulgence in eating. In sex. Overindulgence in everything. And, Roger, I am fully convinced of this: Overindulgence in any and *every* abuse is cumulative. It stacks up. It adds up . . ."

"Wow! That's heavy, man. Heavy!"

"I'm not finished, Roger. I don't think AIDS just *happens* to somebody in a month or so of abuse. Or a year. Or ten years. In my opinion the kind of abuse we're talking about—depending upon the severity— may take twenty years. Or thirty years. But there will come a day of reckoning."

"What about children, then? And babies? Some of

them get AIDS. How do they get it?"

I shook my head. "Roger, many children . . . and babies have been impacted from the moment of conception. Some even before conception, by the abusive living of their mothers. And their fathers. With drugs, with their partying. Their negative thinking. These babies have been immune suppressed in the womb, in the amniotic fluid. And then, shortly after birth they're filled with vaccines and innoculations . . . and *all of those factors* suppress the immune system."

Beads of sweat were forming on Roger's forehead, but he was hanging on every word I was saying.

"And, now, Roger, I'm going to give it to you straight: Your body has had it. You are facing your day of reckoning. That's the reason you've got AIDS. And if we don't find a way to reverse the damage you're going to die."

I reached across the table and grabbed his hand. "I'm sorry, Roger. You don't know how sorry I am. And you don't know how hard it's been for me to lay this on you. But those are the facts."

He swallowed hard. He looked at his half empty cup of coffee like it was poison. He shoved it away from him so violently that it spilled. His answered me in a husky voice. "Bob, in my heart I know you're right. And I'm scared. I'm really scared." He looked at me like a frightened, sick child. "Bob . . . do you honestly think I've got a chance? I mean a chance of making it?"

With my finger I traced a pattern in the spilled coffee. "I don't know, Roger. I honestly don't know. But I believe we've crossed the first hurdle . . ."

"What do you mean?"

"The first hurdle, I think, was at least intellectually determining the cause of AIDS. The second one—and it's been a tough one for both of us—has been for you to face up to the fact that you, Roger, and you alone are responsible for your condition . . . right?"

He nodded miserably.

"And the third one, which I'm dedicating my full attention to is this: Is it possible to reverse the immune system damage? I don't know if it's possible. All the medical evidence I've got at my disposal tells me no. But, *I don't believe it*! You're a relatively young man, Roger. And if you'll be my guinea pig, my laboratory rat, I believe there's a slim chance that we can do what's never been done before. At least to my knowledge . . ."

"Prevent AIDS from killing its intended victim?"

"That's right. With your full cooperation—and I do mean *full cooperation*—I'm going to give it all I've got. Are you with me? All the way?"

Roger held out both hands and gripped mine. Both of us had tears in our eyes. "I pledge myself totally to help you in every way, Bob," he said. "I won't question anything you do. I'll just do it . . ."

I grinned. "Beginning right now?"

"Beginning right now."

"With coffee?"

Roger grimaced. "With coffee. With God's help, this is the last cup of coffee I'll ever drink. The last caffeine I'll ever taste. I am with you all the way!"

CHAPTER TEN

True to his word, Roger kicked his caffeine addiction. Cold turkey. But, true to my predictions, it wasn't easy. In fact, it nearly killed him. His ordeal turned out to be life-threatening for him and "profession-threatening" for me.

I didn't hear from Roger all the next day, but my bedside phone buzzed at three A.M. the following morning. I had a woman about to deliver in the hospital so I was halfway expecting a call. I picked it up on the first buzz. At the sound of panic in Roger's voice, I sat bolt upright.

"I can't do it, Bob. I can't do it!" I recognized his voice immediately, but his words were so slurred that I could hardly make out what he was saying.

"Can't do what, Roger? What can't you?"

"Kick it cold . . . coffee . . . I've got to have a cup. I think I'm dying!"

"Hold on, Roger," I said. "I'll take the call in the next room . . . don't go away. Hold on." I put the phone on hold and struggled into my robe.

Mary sat up. "What's wrong?"

"I don't know for sure. Try to go back to sleep.

Okay?" She snuggled down and I covered up her shoulder.

"Let me know, Bob. Okay?"

"I will."

When I picked up the phone in my office, I could hear what I thought was Roger's teeth chattering. "Okay, Roger . . . I'm here. Give me the whole story."

"I'm sick, Bob. Awful sick. I don't think I can do it . . . I just can't do it. Help me, Bob. Help me. Please help me."

"Where are you?"

"I'm in my room. Haven't left it since you left me here."

I heard retching sounds and moved the receiver from my ear till they stopped. "Roger! Are you alright?"

"I don't know, Bob. I don't think so . . . Bob, you've got to help me. Please help me. Give me something for this . . . for God's sake, give me something. I think I'm dying."

I made a quick decision. I couldn't let him down. "Roger, hold on, buddy. I've got to call the hospital. I'll be there as soon as I can make it. Okay?"

"Please hurry, Bob. Please hurry . . ."

"Unlock your door, Roger. I'll come right in."

I called the hospital and asked the floor nurse about my patient. "She's alright, Doctor. Not much change. I don't think she'll deliver before morning."

I gave her Roger's number. "I'll be there in about fifteen minutes," I said. "I'll call you before I leave there. If you need me sooner, just beep me."

I dressed hurriedly, whispered my plans to Mary and wheeled out of the driveway. The night was cold and the stars were bright. "What have I done?" I asked myself. "Maybe Roger's too weak to be taken off coffee. God help him . . ."

With books, papers and castoff clothes scattered, Roger's room was a shambles. Shoes on, partially disrobed, his coat pulled up to his chin, Roger was stretched out on top of his bed. A two-thirds empty whiskey bottle was on the bedside stand. His face, pale and drawn, in stark contrast to a twenty-four hour patchy stubble, if Roger not been trembling so violently, I could easily have taken him for dead.

I carefully picked my way around the spots where Roger had missed the wastebasket and had thrown up on the carpet. The stench was almost more than I could handle. My stomach muscles tightened in revulsion.

Roger's eyes were pinched shut and his lips were moving, but no sound came. I threw a towel over the messes on the carpet and carefully made my way over to the bed. Roger made no move as I sat down beside him on the bed and picked up his limp wrist. His pulse was weak, fast and thready; his breathing shallow and irregular; his skin cold and clammy. Apparently unable to cope with caffeine withdrawal, Roger had taken a few drinks, gotten dead drunk and passed out.

The telephone was on the bed beside him, the receiver off the hook. I hung up, got a dial tone and called the hospital. Within an hour, without having regained consciousness, Roger was strapped in a bed in ICU.

"I shouldn't have left Roger alone," I berated myself. Now, when (or if) he survives, in addition to his battle with AIDS and caffeine addiction, my friend and patient could be faced with yet another serious problem.

At five-thirty my female patient delivered a healthy

boy child. No complications. When I left the new mother and father they were ecstatic with joy. Then, showered and ready for the day, I called Mary at six. "I'm at the hospital," I told her. "So is Roger. I've got him in ICU . . ."

"Intensive care? What happened? Is he alright?"

"He was unconscious . . . passed out . . . when I got to his room. I could do nothing for him in the hotel . . ."

"But, what happened?"

"Honey, I'm not sure. He may simply have gotten drunk . . ." I felt weak and sick at my stomach, from the stress and lack of sleep. Along with my concern for Roger.

"When will you be home?" Mary asked. "You sound exhausted."

"I am. I need to make rounds. That'll take about two hours. Fortunately I don't have surgery this morning. Then I've got to attend to Roger. I hope I can be there around nine-thirtyish."

"Okay, Bob. I'll have a nice breakfast for you." She paused, then, "Bob, I love you very much. Please take good care of yourself. Okay? For me?"

"I promise, Mary. I love you too."

Roger didn't regain consciousness until late in the afternoon. "Dr. Cochran is slightly disoriented," the ICU nurse told me when she called me at my office. "He's begging for coffee," she said. "Should I give it to him?"

"No. No coffee. No stimulants of any kind. How are his vital signs?"

"Within acceptable limits. Pulse 95. Respiration 20. Blood pressure elevated. Last reading, 150/100."

"And his EKG?"

"I'm keeping a good eye on that."

"Thanks. Call me if there's any change."

Later that evening I saw Roger. He was conscious and seemed to be in good spirits, considering. "What happened?" he asked.

"You'll have to tell me," I said. "I got to your room about twenty minutes after you called. Found you unconscious. I called the ambulance. And here you are. How do you feel?"

"Worse than when the hospital roof fell on me when Charley bombed us in Saigon." He looked rather sheepish. "Sorry to have caused you so much trouble."

I squeezed his arm. "You're my patient. Remember. Patients are *supposed* to need attention, aren't they?"

"I guess so. But not at midnight . . ."

"Three-thirty a.m.," I corrected.

"Oh, no, Bob. I am sorry."

"It's alright. At least I think so. Seems that you're going to be out of ICU in the morning. . . . Now, Roger, feel like telling me all about it?"

He nodded. "I guess so. I'm really ashamed. Well, it all began right after you dropped me off at my room yesterday . . . I guess it was yesterday . . ."

"Day *before* yesterday."

"Oh. Well, anyway, I felt like I'd been pulled through a knothole. So I went downstairs to the restaurant. Without thinking, I ordered myself a cup of coffee. When it came I even picked it up—habit, y'know—before I remembered. Then I set it down . . . didn't even taste it. But, Bob, that coffee *smelled* so good . . ."

"Then what?"

"I told the waiter to take it away. Tried to explain to him. But I could tell he didn't understand what I was trying to tell him. By that time my stomach was tied up in knots . . . so I went to my room . . ."

"What time was that?" I broke in.

"Not sure. Oh, yes, around five-thirty. So I turned on the TV and watched part of the news. Then, twice within a 30-minute segment they advertised coffee. I couldn't stand it, so I snapped off the TV and tried to read. Couldn't keep my attention on anything. So I went for a walk . . ."

"Where'd you go?"

"Finally ended up in a movie. Watched about half of it. Don't even remember the name of it. Then, Bob, I just *had* to have a cup of coffee . . . just had to. I'm sorry."

"And you did?"

"Yeah . . . I did. Broke my promise to you. But, Bob, it seemed like I was coming apart at the seams. Like a bunch of springs inside of me were jumping around. I couldn't hold my hand steady. Sick at my stomach. Trembling. Nervous. Palpitations of the heart. All that . . ."

I just raised my eyebrows, but didn't respond.

"I know, I know. You warned me. And with my background, I should have known. But, Bob, I've never known anybody that's experienced anything more than discomfort when they kicked coffee. But what I had was more than discomfort. It was terrible! It was about like coming off hard drugs. It really shook me. Jolted me. Y'know?"

I nodded. "Yes, I know. I've seen quite a few lately. Many of them pretty difficult. But, Roger, you've got to remember your condition's not exactly tip-top right now. Anyway, you felt like you were coming apart. So you had a cup of coffee. Then what?"

"Surprised me. That one cup didn't help. Seemed to make it worse. I started to order another one . . .

but, then, I didn't. Then I got angry . . ."

"Angry? At me for telling you to kick the habit?"

"No, not you, Bob. Well, yes. But just for a minute or so. I was mostly angry at myself for being so weak. I knew that AIDS had made me weak . . . but I still thought I had some moral fiber left. At least enough to keep my word to my doctor . . ."

He looked up at me apologetically and impulsively grabbed my hand. ". . . and my best friend. I really mean it, Bob. I don't think I've ever had a friend like you . . ."

I gripped his hand. "You've been a good buddy, Roger. Go on with your story."

"So, I said to myself, 'I've got to get through this . . . somehow. So I'll just have a drink or two and go to sleep.' " He shook his head. "I can't handle it like I used to, Bob. Just took a couple of drinks, maybe three, and I got sicker than I've ever been . . . never used to get sick when I drank. I threw up . . ."

He took a deep breath. "Guess I made a mess of my room, didn't I?"

"Yep, quite a mess, Roger. Go on."

"It seemed like I had the DT's or something. Like my whole body was rebelling. Got the shakes. Couldn't walk straight. I was so cold I thought I'd die. And, Bob, this is funny . . . well, not really funny . . . but when I woke up again, I thought if I didn't get a cup of coffee inside of me that I would die and go to hell . . ."

"That's when you called me?"

"I guess so. I don't remember very clearly." Roger looked up at me with a pleading expression. "What do you think, Doc. Am I going to . . . to, make it?"

"Sure thing, Roger," I said, with more conviction that I was feeling. "Sure you'll make it."

Roger didn't look convinced. "Doc, I've used that same tone of voice on hundreds of patients." He fixed me with eyes that were steadier now. "You're not sure, are you?"

"Look, Roger," I said, "can't we talk about this in the morning? You'll be more rested . . ."

"No, Bob, not tomorrow. Right now. I'd like some sort of an idea where you think I stand. What do you think happened to me? And do you think I'm going to make it. I mean, am I going to die? Or live?"

"Roger, you're really putting me on the spot, you know that. I'm not God. And I don't know all the answers . . ."

"Look, Bob, I *know* all those kind of beside-manner answers. I'm a doctor, too. Remember? But right now I'm the patient. And I had a close call. Honestly, what do you think my chances are?"

I cleared my throat. "Roger, as near as I can tell, you had a mixed reaction of some kind. Your immune system is all messed up, you know that. The attempt to break with caffeine cold turkey may have been too much. On top of that your bout with the bottle compounded things . . ."

Roger broke in impatiently. "Bob, I *know* all that. I know it. I guess what I really need from you is your assurance that you're going to stick with me . . . stick with me, and see it to the end. One way or the other." He finished lamely. "Yeah, that is what I want, Bob. You're assurances . . . honest assurances. Is that too much to ask?"

I looked around me before I spoke. "Roger, the ICU is hardly the place to be having such a heavy doctor-patient discussion."

"I know that, too, Bob. But last night I came face to face with my mortality. And I realized that I could die. That I *might* die. And that you, Doctor Bob, *you* are the only viable link I've got with life . . ."

"C'mon, Roger . . ." I began.

"Bob, just listen. You and I both know that's the truth. If I mess up with you, I've had it. And that scares me. Bob, to tell you the truth, I'm not sure I can do it . . ."

"Do what?"

"Kick coffee . . . or AIDS, or . . . or anything." Tears began rolling down Roger's sunken cheeks. "But, Bob, like I've told you before, I don't want to die." He gripped my hand and held on as though his life depended upon it. "Bob, will you give me another chance? Please?"

Perhaps for the very first time, I realized that Roger's physical and emotional reserves were gone. He was at the bottom. And that he was walking a tight rope—between reality and unreality, between life and death—that I was holding on to one end. And the other end wasn't in Roger's hands. It was in God's hands. This was a critical moment for Roger.

I did not dare let him lose faith, not for a moment, because it might prove fatal. In that millisecond between Roger's plea and my answer, I wondered about my own professionalism. My own emotional and spiritual strength. I saw clearly the fragility of the human spirit, and that Roger's was unable to withstand even the slightest additional strain.

At that moment I knew that I was Roger's link with life, and that the answer I now gave him would either save him or destroy him. "Oh, God . . . let it be right," I prayed under my breath.

I leaned over my friend and gripped his bony shoulders with my hands. Gripped them until he winced in pain. "Roger . . . Roger . . ." I began, then was overcome with emotion. "Roger, we've been through a lot together, haven't we?"

He nodded, his eyes fixed on mine as though that visual contact meant his life. He whispered a hoarse, "Yes, Bob . . ."

"Do you remember that night in that Saigon bar . . . the night those two drunk Marines were trying to kill me. Remember?"

"Yeah, I remember. They said you'd let their buddy die. And they were going to make you pay . . . I remember."

"Those guys were big. And mean. And drunk enough to follow through on what they said. They fully intended to kill me . . ."

Roger nodded. "I remember."

"Then, suddenly, there came this roar from the background—and a huge grizzly bear of a man grabbed those two bruisers—and tossed them over the bar . . . like they'd been rag dolls. Remember that night, Roger?"

He just shook his head and mouthed, "Yeah."

"Roger, I vowed that night, that come hell or high water, if I ever had the opportunity to repay you for saving my life . . . whatever it took, I'd do it. Remember me telling you that?"

Tears splashed on Roger's pillow. He nodded.

"Well, buddy, now's my chance to make my promise to you good. You don't ever have to ask me for another chance. Maybe you blew it, and maybe you didn't. We'll never know. We'll never know how it was that your human weakness and alcohol and caffeine and AIDS conspired to kill you . . ."

I released my hold and stood up straight. "But, Roger . . . I am telling you, just like I told you that night in Saigon . . . *whatever it takes*—whatever. I'm not going to let you go or let you down. I will stay with you to the end. Okay?"

He reached up and gripped my hand. "Okay, Bob. Okay."

"This has been an awful night for you, Roger. You could have died. It's been an awful night for me, too, in a different way."

"What do you mean?"

I took a deep breath. "Tonight, while I was waiting for that baby to be born, waiting for a new life to come into the world. I was thinking about life. About you. I was thinking about me and my life: about medicine, my profession. I was thinking about drugs. I was thinking about the damage they have done. And I was wondering if I had the intestinal fortitude—the guts—to hold the line . . . against, well, call it medical tradition, to the point where I could see a real breakthrough . . ."

"You can do it, Bob," Roger said. "You can do it."

I nodded. "After tonight, I believe I can. I'm not sure that I've helped you all I could. I thought I had. But I'm not sure I've given it all I've got. But, Roger, God helping me, I'm going to do it. No, better yet, *we'll* do it. Okay, buddy?"

He nodded. "Okay, buddy." He blew his nose loudly and gave me that all-familiar lopsided grin. "And now, Doctor, I think you've better leave. Your patient needs to rest. And now, Bob, I think I can rest. G'night."

I think Roger was asleep before I left ICU.

CHAPTER ELEVEN

It took about a week for Roger's condition to stabilize
to the point that he could go home. This time,
though, I engaged a private nurse to check in with
him two or three times a day. As I anticipated, Roger
objected. "Look, I don't need a babysitter. I can man-
age . . ."

I grinned. "Sure you can. Like you did before."

"That was a low blow, Bob. But is a nurse necessary?"

"Roger, face it, you're not out of woods yet. You've
got a long way to go. A long, *long* ways to go. We've
just begun to scratch the surface. In addition to
AIDS, we're still working on that coffee addiction."

"I can handle it."

"Roger, the answer is: I'm your doctor. And if I
have to pull rank on you, I'm going to do it. Period.
The nurse stays. How long she stays depends on
you."

"Okay, okay. You win. Sorry to be stubborn."

"I'm going to be very pointed with you, Roger. It's
clear that sometimes I may have to protect you from
yourself . . ."

He winced, but nodded.

"Have you ever taken AZT?"

"You mean azidothymidine? The experimental drug for AIDS?"

"Right, trade name is Retrovir. Have you taken it?"

Roger shook his head. "No, Bob," his tone bitter. "I tried to get in the program. Didn't make it. Why do you ask?"

"The drug's got certain side effects, such as ane-mia. And if I'm going to be effective in working with you, I've got to know everything that's going on in your body . . . and in your life. Right?"

He drew a long breath. "Right."

"Another question: Are you taking any drugs or medications of any kind?"

I could almost see the struggle going on within Roger. On the one hand, I am certain he wanted to cooperate fully; but on the other hand, he was fearful of losing his autonomy if he told all. After a short pause, he nodded. "Yes. I'm taking Miltown. But only when I get tense or upset . . ."

"And that's all?"

He nodded. "Do you want me to give that up too?"

I shook my head. "Not now. Or not yet. I don't want to try and move too fast. Later, yes . . . but, Roger . . .?"

He recognized the question in my voice. "But, what?"

"We've got to work as a team. If you hold back from me—anything—it's like an attorney trying to protect a client without knowing the whole truth. You know that."

He answered slowly. "Bob, I know that. But I've been such an independent guy . . . doctor . . . for so long, it's really hard to switch places. And become the patient. You understand?"

"Probably not. I can only imagine how difficult it must be. I'll try to be sensitive to that . . . but there will be times when I might have to pull rank on you. And when I do, Roger, I've got to have your full co-operation."

He stuck out his hand. Solemnly he said, "I'll give you my word again. You might have to remind me again. But, I agree in principle. And in practice. Well, I'll do my very best . . ."

"That's all I can ask." I turned to go, then turned back. "And, Roger, let me tell you this, I *am* proud of you. I believe we've made a good beginning. The nurse will check with me each time she sees you. But I'd like for you to call me every day, too. Will you do that?"

"Yes, Bob, I will." He paused. "And . . . Bob, if it means anything to you, I lit a couple of candles for you last night."

"Thanks, Roger. It does mean something. Thanks."

A few days later when he called, he reported, "I don't the have the shakes anymore. I'm still weak. Guess I have to get used to that . . . at least until . . ." He left the ending of that sentence unfinished. "I still feel like I need my morning caffeine fix. And I've still got those headaches . . ."

"Good going, Roger. Good beginning. Say, it's about time for you and me to have lunch again. Can you come in tomorrow? Same time and place?"

"Okay. See you there."

The next day before we ordered, I said, "Roger, this is your doctor talking. Okay?"

He raised his eyebrows. "Another prescription? What is it this time?"

"Today I want you to have a salad. No steak. And

no French fries. Alright?"

"Sure. But, why? I thought today you'd let me celebrate."

"We are celebrating. But we're going to do it sanely. Last time we ate here I saw you practically cover everything with salt. So, beginning today, let's cut out the salt. Okay?"

Roger shrugged, but I knew he wasn't pleased. "Are you trying to take all the fun from my life?"

"No, sir, Roger. What I'm trying to do is give your life back to you so you can really live, really have fun. The last time we checked your blood pressure it was way too high. So, all we're doing is trying to eliminate the major culprit." I grinned at him. "And, *Doctor* Cochran, how many times have you said the same thing to one of your patients?"

"Touche, Bob. Okay, it'll be tough. Because I do love my salt. But you're the doctor."

Roger's mein was meditative, which I respected. Neither of us spoke again until our salads came. Finally he said, "Bob, I really do appreciate what you're doing for me. And from personal experience, I know how frustrating it is for a patient to kick and complain. So, I promise again that I will obey all your instructions. I won't cheat. Not even once."

"And, like I said, Roger, I'm proud of you. Because, buddy, I believe we can, *and we will* lick the thing that's trying its best to lick you. Right?"

"Right on!"

Along with most medical doctors, my training in preventive medicine was anything but strong. My orientation was more in the curing end, than the preventing end. And though this trend may be changing somewhat, I know from experience that most doctors have got a long ways to go in the preventing business.

So you can see that I was walking a tight rope, and (to mix metaphors) trying to wend my way through a complex maze composed of academic medical training on one hand and intuitive patient care on the other. I was trying to move carefully and slowly, but not too slowly, so as not to make any bad mistakes.

For me, and I'm sure for Roger, progress (mostly negligible, often none) was agonizingly slow. But I had to remind myself that I was breaking trail. Because, at this point, on the course I had set out for myself, there simply was nobody else to follow. I was reading everything I could get hold of that offered any hope or encouragement. (Such material was practically non-existent.) I was also doing lots of thinking. And, incidentally, I was doing my share of praying.

I was so intensely involved with Roger's case (sometimes *tensely*) that I was finding it more and more difficult to sleep. I knew I was on the verge of something, but after the initial breakthrough it seemed that I had reached an impasse. I knew that the mere fact that I *knew* I was right made little difference if I couldn't prove it in practice.

Now, though, I had something to work with that I hadn't had before: I had Roger as a "laboratory rat" with which to "experiment." I winced at the word, but I knew it was true. What I would do with Roger—when I could determine just what to do— would be amounting to the same kind of experiments I had done with Adam and Eve while I was in high school.

Mary and I had gone to bed early and she had dropped off within seconds. But not I. For days now I'd been troubled by a nagging half-thought that had hovered just outside my mental grasp. But it kept eluding me. The more I struggled to snare it and to bring it into full focus, the more elusive it became.

Finally I gave up. Like a fetus—when it is fully matured and ready for delivery—I reasoned, will have its natural way (and nothing can prevent it), so will this elusive thought when it's ready to be "borned."

Lying with my fingers laced together behind my head, staring into the darkness, I heard the down-stairs clock chime every half hour. When it chimed twelve and I was no more asleep than when I'd re-tired, I quietly slid out of bed, fumbled into my robe and tiptoed downstairs to my study. Restless, unable to concentrate, I paced the floor . . .

Why wouldn't that undeveloped thought reach full term and be born? I knew it had something to do with Roger. As did most of my thoughts these days. I paused in my pacing to glance over my stack of un-read AMA journals. But nothing held my attention.

Unbidden, a line from Edgar Allen Poe came to mind:

> "Once upon a midnight dreary, while I pondered, weak and weary,
> Over many a quaint and curious volume of forgotten lore. . . ."

Forgotten lore. For some reason decipherable only to doctors of the mind, those two words began to ring in my ears. Forgotten lore . . . forgotten lore. Then it came to me, the thought that had eluded me all night. Somewhere in my forgotten, unread books there was an out-of-print book that had to do with the subject of abusive lifestyles. At least I thought it did. I had picked it up at a used bookstore a couple of years ago and had never read it.

"What *is* the title of that book?" I asked myself. "And who is the author?"

I knew it had something to do with toxic poisoning. But not the newer poisoning due to toxic waste dumping. Toxic foods. Toxic lifestyles. I turned on all my office lights and started a systematic search for that book of "forgotten lore." I became aware of my heart pounding in eagerness . . .

Ten minutes later I came across it. The hardback cover was still in excellent condition. At the time I purchased it, I remember thinking that some doctor had bought it, read it, disagreed with the author's premise, and discarded it. I had already purchased a score of books that day, but because this particular book still looked good, I thought it might be a good one to add to my library.

Toxemia Explained was the title, written by J. H. Tilden, M.D. My fingers were trembling as I opened to the Preface.

"From time immemorial," the book began, "man has looked for a savior; and, when not looking for a savior, he is looking for a cure. . . . Instead of buying, begging, or stealing a cure, *it is better to stop building disease*. Disease is man's own building."

I put a marker in the book and closed my eyes. I remember having read those words when I found the book. Mary and I had been spending a few days on a holiday in San Francisco. Fortunately for me, she shares my love for books. And at some time on any of our excursions we invariably ended up in used book stores.

"Mary, listen to this," I said, and read to her the words I had just read. She looked up from her own stack of dusty books and smiled. "It makes sense . . ."

93

"Makes sense? Mary, it's stupid! Disease attacks people. People don't make their own diseases. Everybody knows that."

She shrugged and laughed. "Well, Bob, don't get all worked up about the book. If you don't like what the author is saying, put it back. You don't have to agree with him, do you?"

I grumbled a little. "Guess you're right." I started to put it back on the shelf. "Well, it's a good-looking book. And it's only a couple of dollars. What's the difference? Might be good for a laugh some day . . ."

So I had carried it home without another look and slid it in between two other books on the subject. My computer memory had locked onto those words and had become the elusive half thought that had evaded me all night. By now I was hungry. I went to the kitchen and got me a banana, then settled back in my favorite reading chair.

There is but a single cause for every disease, Tilden was saying. And that cause is toxemia.

"Law and order pervades the universe, the same yesterday, today and forever, and is the same from star-dust to mind—from electron to mind. Toxemia explains how the universal law operates in health and disease. . . . If wrong eating is persisted in, the acid fermentation first irritates the mucous membrane of the stomach; the irritation become inflamation, then ulceration, then thickening and hardening, which ends in cancer at last.

"The medical world is struggling to find the cause of cancer. It is the distal end of an inflammatory process whose proximal beginning may be any irritation. . . ."

A prayer of thankfulness arose to my lips. "Thank

94

God. Thank God. I believe this is another missing piece . . ."

For the first time since I had interned, I read all night long. And when morning came, much too soon to suit me, I had completely read Tilden's small book. From that small beginning, my medical practice was irrevocably changed. I set out that morning to reorient my mind to healing instead of drugging and prevention instead of cure.

Not that I had all the answers. I did not, and to date, I do not have them all. But the light that had gone on within me a few days ago was now shining brighter than ever. Prior to the relocating and reading of this book, I had *believed* that I knew the causes of AIDS, now, deep within me, *I knew*.

Though with Roger, it was abundantly clear that time was of the essence, and we had none to waste, I was certain that I now would be able to determine a course of action that could reverse the course of the disease that was killing him and return him to a perfect state of wellness.

CHAPTER TWELVE

Altogether, I had poured more than twenty years of my life into the medical profession. And I was proud to be a physician. Yet, I was beginning to have difficulty reconciling some of the conflicting reports in the media regarding the efficacy of medical treatment.

On the one hand I would read glowing reports from the National Cancer Institute regarding the progress being made in the war against cancer, such as the letter to the Editor of the *Los Angeles Times*, dated March 21, 1987. In part the NCI doctor wrote, "The effectiveness of existing cancer treatments is very real, and much progress has been made based on basic and clinical research."

And on the other hand a well-documented major article in *The New England Journal of Medicine*, dated May 8, 1986 indicated that between the years of 1950 to 1982, "In the United States, these years were associated with increases in the number of deaths from cancer. . . . *we are losing the war against cancer.*"

Concerning the same subject and the same period of time, Bob DeBragga, Executive Director of Project

CURE made the statement in his newsletter that "The nation is losing the War Against Cancer because the many effective nutritional and other non-toxic preventatives and treatments for cancer are being completely ignored by the medical establishment."

Nutritional and other non-toxic preventatives . . . I filed that statement away in my mind for future cogitation.

If such opposing views and statements regarding cancer-related information were being reported and bandied about by the experts, could I expect anything different, more reliable or more accurate concerning AIDS? The answer to me seemed clear: It was not possible.

The more I read and carefully examined the literature, the more clear the difference between the reporting on cancer and AIDS was becoming: For some reason as yet unclear to me, with cancer it seemed important not to tell all the truth, which, because of its burgeoning death toll, was extremely negative. I couldn't overlook the nearly *one half million* deaths from cancer each year, with the number steadily rising!

Epidemic figures if ever I heard them, but they are played down.

In comparison, I took note of the miniscule numbers of AIDS victims—since 1980, fewer than 40,000, only one half of which were fatal. Compared to cancer and heart disease, this figure could hardly be considered epidemic.

With cancer, I realized, the statistics were being *played down*. But with AIDS, the statistics were being *played up*! Why the difference? I asked myself. It was evident that practically every newspaper, magazine and TV news broadcast in the nation is force-feeding

AIDS "news" to an increasingly panicked populace on a daily, almost hourly basis.

Why is this? I again asked myself.

I set myself to find out. What I learned is very disturbing.

I began to total the numbers, and was appalled. Literally billions of dollars are being appropriated *each year*, purportedly in a search for an AIDS vaccine. I say *purportedly*, because, as I weighed and sifted all the media output, I became angry at what I was beginning to believe is a fruitless, smoke screen witch hunt for a "cure" that does not exist.

My growing skepticism was buttressed as I read the following statement from "Health Freedom News" (May 1986): "In the past 10 years alone, during which the American Cancer Society has collected more than $1 *billion* from the American public, and the cancer industry has collected over *$10 billion* each year, deaths from cancer *climbed 12 percent!*"

I also learned from a fellow physician, Sidney M. Wolfe, in his excellent book *Pills That Don't Work*, of 610 drugs used by the orthodox medical establishment *which have either never been tested or have been tested and found totally worthless*. I now realize that billions of these ineffective, worthless drugs continue to be sold by the orthodox medical establishment—of which I am a part—to patients who are in search of miracles that never happen.

Obviously these statements related to cancer. But we are doubtless experiencing a corollary in the AIDS phenomenon. I asked myself, "Does all of this represent an exercise in futility?" And I was reminded of my wife's sage observation, "Perhaps they are looking for a cure in the wrong places."

I was even more ready to agree with her quip when

I read the article in *The New York Times*, March 18, 1987, in which appeared the statement: "Despite the size and speed of the global research effort, a proven vaccine does not appear likely for five or ten years, *perhaps not before the next century.* . . . Scientists are not even sure whether it will be possible to develop a vaccine against the AIDS virus."

I told Mary—I couldn't tell my colleagues—"My faith in my chosen profession is being shaken." It left me with an uneasy, troubled feeling. To whom could I turn for the truth? Dr. Mendelsohn? Dr. John Tilden?

Maybe Tilden's book held more truth than I realized.

Roger's voice on the telephone sounded excited. "Bob! Bob, have you heard of Harvey Diamond?"

He caught me off guard. "Harvey Diamond? Should I know him? The name sounds a little familiar . . ."

"You should know the name, Bob. He and his wife wrote the book, *Fit For Life*. It's a best seller."

"Oh, yes. I've heard of the book. A couple of my patients have asked me about it. Why do you ask?"

"I just saw Harvey and his wife on TV. And they look great, Bob. Really great. I'm going down to get their book."

"Well, okay, Roger . . . but don't do anything drastic. Okay? I mean, we've gotten a good start . . ."

"I promise, Bob. You've got my word on that. I'll tell you about it. See ya."

I shrugged as I hung up the phone. *Just a flash in the pan*, I thought, and dismissed the whole conversation. I remembered the book now. A couple of doctors and I discussed the book at the hospital one morning. At least they discussed it and I listened.

"It's a dangerous book!" Dan Halley said. Dan's one of the best internists I know, and I personally value his judgment. "I think Harvey Diamond should be charged with practicing medicine without a license!"

Tom Holmes agreed, but he put it even stronger than Halley. Dr. Tom is the crusty president of a local AMA, and a strong advocate of the inviolability of the AMA. "The guy should be locked up!" he growled. "He'll have people trying to treat themselves, and they'll end up sicker than ever. Or dead."

"What's Diamond saying?" I asked, looking from one to the other of the two doctors.

"He says the most important food a person can eat is fruit," Dan said, pouring himself another cup of the cafeteria's strong, black coffee. "He says Americans are eating too much protein, and that eating too much causes all kinds of diseases . . ."

"Such as?" I asked.

"You name it. Heart disease, high blood pressure, cancer, gout, arthritis . . ." Holmes said.

"And osteoporosis," Dan added.

"Sheer stupidity," Dr. Tom said.

"Diamond talks like he's an authority on internal medicine," Dan said.

"Where did he get his training?" I asked.

"From some institution in Texas, I think they call it the American College of Health Science. Something like that," Dan said. "I've never heard of it."

Dr. Tom muttered something I didn't understand and motioned with his coffee cup to the waiter. I could tell this conversation was going nowhere.

I shoved back my chair. "I haven't read the book," I said, "so there's not much I can add." I slapped them both on the shoulders. "And upon the recommendation of you two worthies, I'm not likely to be reading it. See you." They were still verbally castigating Diamond when I left them.

After Roger hung up, I momentarily thought of phoning him back and warning him about Diamond's book. But then I shrugged. "He's a big boy," I thought "and he'll soon see the weaknesses in the man's philosophy." With that I dismissed the whole matter.

During the winter months I was getting my share of colds, sore throats and flu patients, and every afternoon my waiting room was filled to overflowing with runny-nosed kids and coughing parents. I treated them as I had always done: with a shot of antibiotics, a prescription for pills, and orders to go home to bed. Paradoxically—despite my growing concern over the dangers of drugs and our drugged society—the incongruity of this action didn't enter my mind.

Though Dr. David's practice was as busy as mine, we still took time for our weekly communication and planning session. "I think I've given a hundred flu shots this week," he said while we waited for our food to come.

I nodded. "So have I. I think Americans take more drugs than they should."

David looked at me strangely. "What do you mean?"

"They take drugs for everything—drugs for colds, drugs for headaches, drugs for depression, drugs for . . ." I took a bite of my sandwich. "What did we ever do before we had all these drugs?"

"Are you suddenly anti-drug, or something?" David asked.

"I guess I am. Too many drugs will kill a person . . ."

"But you *give* drugs, Bob. You give shots. You give prescriptions. We both do. Is there anything wrong with that?"

I started to take a bite, then put my sandwich down. "Yes, there is, David. We've got drugs in everybody's home. In every woman's purse . . . in every businessman's brief case, and every kid's locker. We see them hawked on every TV show. It's no wonder kids take to drugs. They're just modelling their elders' behavior, that's all."

"I've never heard you talk like this, Bob. If you're so set against drugs, why do you prescribe them? And give them?"

Not until that moment did the incongruity of my actions hit me. "That's a good question, David," I said slowly. "And the answer is—I don't know."

I left the restaurant that day with a growing tight knot in my stomach. People were taking drugs because I gave them drugs! Women were taking tranquilizers because I prescribed them. Overweight men and woman were taking diuretics because I advised them to do so. Girls were taking the Pill because they asked for them—and by my overt act of prescribing them, I made the implied statement that I thought they were doing the right thing.

"My God," I told Janine that afternoon, "We doctors are as much involved in the drug abuse problem as the pusher on the street . . ."

"No, Doctor Bob," she tried to console me, "you're not. You are dispensing legal drugs. They're selling illegal drugs . . ."

I shook my head, "The end result is the same.

We're both selling drugs. And drugs—legal or illegal—are killing the people. Killing the parents. Killing the children. Killing the young people. No, Janine, I can't rationalize my way out of this one. In a way I'm no better than a legalized drug pusher."

I reached for a book on my desk, "A case in point. This came recently, free, from the American Academy of Pediatrics . . ." I handed the 140-page publication that was titled, "Management of Pediatric Practice."

"Yes, I saw it when it came in," Janine said.

"I knew you did. But did you read the form letter that came with it?"

She shook her head.

"The letter says, 'This publication is provided under *an educational grant* made possible by Wyeth Laboratories.' " I looked up. "Do you know what Wyeth Laboratories manufactures?"

"I'm not sure."

"They manufacture infant formula and antibiotics."

"I don't understand what you're getting at," Janine said.

"Just this: within the book there is a self-serving section devoted to how the doctor should entertain 'pharmaceutical representatives,' in other words, drug salesmen. In part, this is what it says, '*Representatives have important information for the pediatrician about pharmaceuticals. . . .*' See what I mean, Janine?"

"Not exactly, because some drugs are *necessary*, aren't they, Doctor Bob?"

"Maybe. Maybe not," I said. "But the point is, actually, I've got two points. First, I think it's wrong for a professional medical organization to allow a drug company to pay for, or print their publications as a means of pushing their drugs.

"Second—something else I don't know what to do about—I think it's quite clear that drugs don't heal diseases. Drugs can't heal anything . . ."

"Then if drugs don't heal, what do they do?"

"Eventually they cause diseases like AIDS . . ."

"Doctor, what are you saying? You can't be serious."

"I'm very serious . . ."

That evening after dinner I pulled out my now familiar copy of *Toxemia Explained*, flipped pages and reread numerous passages I had underlined. "Medical science is founded on a false premise," Tilden had written, "namely, that disease is caused by extraneous influences, and that drugs are something that cures. . . . Medical science is built around the idea that disease can be cured when the right drug is found. . . ."

I had always been taught and had believed, that diseases were "caused" by forces outside the patient. And Tilden was saying, "So-called disease is nature's effort at eliminating the toxins from the blood. All so-called diseases are crises of toxemia. When nerve energy is dissipated from any cause—physical or mental excitement or bad habits—the body becomes enervated, when enervated elimination is checked, causing a retention of toxin in the blood, or toxemia. This accumulation of toxin when once established will continue until nerve energy is restored *by removing the causes*."

But what about the germ theory? I wondered.

As though in anticipation of my question, Tilden had written, "Germs and other so-called causes may be discovered in the course of pathological development, but they are accidental, coincidental, or at most auxiliary or, *obiter dicta* (a legal term meaning, 'having no bearing upon the case in question').

"Disease is perverted health. Any influence that lowers nerve-energy becomes disease producing. Disease cannot be its own cause; neither can it be its own cure."

Who was J. H. Tilden? I asked myself. Who was this man who was speaking so directly to my troubled soul in such a timely manner? The book's brief biography of Dr. John H. Tilden told me that he was himself the son of a doctor. The younger Tilden started his practice of medicine at Nokomis, Illinois, then later moved to Denver, where he was in active practice until his death in September of 1940.

Early in his practice, Dr. Tilden began to question the use of medicine to cure illness. (I was taking special note of this section.) His extensive reading, especially of medical studies from European medical schools, and his own thinking led him to the conclusion that *there should be some way to live so as not to build disease*. Practicing with that philosophy, from the beginning of his practice in Denver, Dr. Tilden used *no medicine* but practiced his theory of ridding the body of toxic poison and then allowing nature to make the cure. He then taught his patients how to live so as not to create a toxic condition and to retain a healthy body free of disease.

Thus, Dr. Tilden practiced medicine for 68 years.

He used *no medicine* . . . no drugs. *Tilden apparently lived what he taught*. I regarded the now closed book in my hand for a long moment and came to a decision. If such a philosophy worked for Dr. Tilden during the first forty years of this century, I reasoned, it can certainly work for me during the last thirteen.

If Tilden could do it, I thought, *then I can do it*!

In that moment I pledged the rest of my professional life to the purpose of teaching my patients how to live so as to maintain their bodies in a constant state of health. At that time I didn't know how I would do this, or even how to begin. But I vowed that I would begin to drug less and less and to counsel more and more.

Though it was late, I dialed Roger Cochran's number. He answered immediately. "Hi, Roger. Bob here. Mind if we talk a few minutes?"

"Okay by me, Doc. What brings you out at such a late hour?"

"I've been reading . . . and thinking. And . . . I think I'm onto something that just might reverse the progress of AIDS . . ."

Roger laughed. "This is funny, Bob. I was just debating about whether I should call you . . ."

"Why? What's up?" I was aware of a new timbre in his voice and it sounded very good.

"Remember Harvey Diamond?"

"I remember."

"Well, I think it's time we talked about his book."

"Why? Is he saying something we should be hearing?"

"You bet your boots . . . and *my* life. Diamond doesn't say anything about AIDS, per se, but he is repeating almost word for word what you told me at the restaurant the other day . . ."

"Which was . . .?"

"Just this: if you're going to enjoy good health, you've got to quit poisoning your body."

"That sounds very good. Did I say that?"

"That's what I thought I heard you say. Anyway, I'd like for you to take a look at this book and advise me. Because I'm beginning to think *we can* reverse the damage that AIDS—that I—have caused to my own body. Did you hear that, Bob, I really am taking full responsibility for my sickness. And with God's help—and yours, not necessarily in that order—I now believe that I, and we are going to turn this thing around!"

"The only thing I can say to that, Roger, is *Amen* and goodnight. We'll meet for lunch tomorrow."

I hung up softly, the new vibrancy of Roger's voice still ringing in my ears.

CHAPTER THIRTEEN

"Just exactly what is AIDS?" Jennifer was asking me.

Jennifer, was a woman I had never met before. She had called my office and arranged with Janine for an appointment with me. Now, seated in my office across the desk from Jennifer, I noted that she was probably in her mid-twenties and quite attractive. Not quite sure how to answer the question, I decided to bid for time. "Why do you ask?" I said.

Though outwardly composed, Jennifer's body language betrayed her nervousness. "Well . . ." she began, apparently thrown off guard, "I've got a friend . . . a . . . a man . . . and, well, he thinks he might have AIDS . . ."

She ended lamely. "And I . . . that is, he wants to know how you can tell if you've got AIDS. I mean, what's it like?" She was twisting her hanky between fingers that were shaking.

"Well, Miss . . ." I began.

"Missus . . ." she corrected me. "Missus Winters. Jennifer Winters . . . But you can call me Jennifer." Unconsciously she began twisting the gold band on her left hand.

I nodded. "Mrs. Winters, uh, Jennifer, AIDS is a very complex disease. And if your husband . . ."

"Friend!" she interjected. "Larry is just a friend . . ."

"Alright. If your friend is concerned about having AIDS, he should come in, or go to his doctor, and be examined." I paused, endeavoring to measure her response.

"Okay . . ." she said slowly. "But what would you—or his doctor—be looking for . . . I mean, what symptoms do people with AIDS have? If you could tell me that . . . then, maybe it would relieve his mind. Don't you agree?"

"Mrs. Winters, excuse me, *Jennifer*, if your friend is really concerned about having AIDS, it would be much better for him to seek medical help than to just imagine . . ."

Now obviously perturbed, the woman started to rise. "Doctor, I thought you might just tell me about AIDS. Can't you just tell me something?"

"Alright, Jennifer," I said. "Just sit down and I'll try to explain to you what AIDS is . . ." As the words left my mouth I suddenly realized that *I myself didn't know exactly what AIDS was or even how to diagnose it in a patient*!

Jennifer Winters sat down and held her breath expectantly. Now the ball was in my court. What would I say? Should I tell Jennifer that, at present, there is no specific laboratory test to detect AIDS? Or that cancer patients receiving chemotherapy, and patients with hepatitis, infectious mononucleosis, and certain other diseases *may* show immunosuppression *similar* to AIDS patients? Should I tell her that some organ transplant patients (who have been given drugs to prevent organ rejection), also evidence similar symptoms as AIDS patients?

Should I get a little bit more technical and tell her that the actual determining factor of a failed immune system is the body's inability to produce adequate white blood cells? Or that prior to the coining of the acronym AIDS, a subnormal count of white blood corpuscles—fewer than 5,000 per cubic millimeter—was called leukocytopenia or lymphocytopenia? But that such a low count is now called AIDS?

I could tell her some or all of those facts. But I decided to tell her none of that. Perhaps I knew that she might not be able to understand what I was saying. Or that all this medical jargon might frighten her.

Instead, I put my elbows on the desk, and in my best patient bedside manner, asked, "Jennifer, do you have any idea what the immune system is?"

She shook her head. "Not really. Except that it's supposed to protect our bodies from getting sick. Is that right?"

I nodded. "You're basically right. When disease-producing organisms or foreign elements get into our bodies they cause problems or infections. The immune system is like an army. When foreign organisms invade our body, our immune system produces antibodies or soldiers that immediately go to battle and destroy the foreign organisms. Is that clear?"

She nodded slowly. "I think so."

"Jennifer, this is a very simplified version, but when the body's immune system—it's protective army—becomes weakened, then it no longer has the power to put up a fight against the invaders. When that happens all kinds of diseases are enabled to develop in the body. And there's nothing to prevent the invaders—the disease-producing organisms—from taking control of the whole territory. The result is AIDS."

The young woman shuddered. She looked at her hands for a long moment. Then slowly, as though in a trance, she withdrew a folded newspaper clipping from her purse and handed it to me. I scanned it quickly.

It was from the *Los Angeles Times*, datelined March 25, 1987, *Washington*, it read: "Surgeon General C. Everett Koop . . . the most visible spokesman on AIDS . . . the *fatal* disease . . ."

When I looked up Jennifer's face had drained of color and I could see her pulse throbbing in her temple. Her hands were no longer busy. They were clasped loosely in her lap. She sighed and the tear-filled eyes she turned upon me were the embodiment of sadness. "Then Larry is going to die," she said flatly.

"Not necessarily," I heard myself saying.

She looked up dully. "But the Surgeon General said . . . he called AIDS fatal . . . didn't he?"

I nodded. "Yes, Jennifer, But that *could* change, couldn't it?"

"I don't know, Doctor. I just don't know." She sighed again. "Well, thank you, Doctor, for taking the time to explain all that to me. I'll be going now . . ." At the door she turned. "How much do I owe you?"

"Nothing, Jennifer. Nothing at all. And, Jennifer . . . if you'd like to have Larry come in . . .?"

She shook her head firmly. "No. He won't come in. He said AIDS victims become guinea pigs for doctors to experiment with. And he said, 'I've got my dignity. I won't become just a guinea pig for some scientist to play with.' That's what he said, Doctor. Then he said that . . ." Her voice choked. "He told me that he'd just, that he'd just . . . stay home and die. Thanks again for talking to me."

And she was gone.

I never heard from Larry. I never saw Jennifer again.

Meanwhile, Roger Cochran was not doing so well. He informed me that he was losing an average of a pound a week. "I just can't eat," he told me. "I don't have an appetite. The very sight of food makes me sick at my stomach." He was no longer salting his food (when he ate) or drinking coffee.

"I'm exhausted all the time," he said. "And it seems that I can't get enough sleep . . . and I'm depressed. Most of the time I think about death and dying . . ."

"Do you read much?" I asked.

"No, Bob, I can hardly stay awake long enough to watch the news on TV. And when I do it makes me even more depressed. I don't know what to do with myself . . . mostly I just lie around all day. And do nothing. I'm vegetating, Bob. Might as well face it— I'm dying . . ."

"Don't say that, Roger. Don't say that! Don't give up!"

He shrugged tiredly. "What's my white count now, Doc?"

I temporized. "I haven't taken it for a few days."

He thrust forth his arm, now well-scarred from "legal" needle tracks. "Take it, Bob. Today. I want to know."

I shook my head. "No need to draw more blood, Roger. It would just weaken you more . . ."

"Then *tell me* what my white count is! Tell me, Bob. I've got a right to know. Tell me."

Though I knew exactly what his count was, I flipped open his chart and glanced over it again. "It's low, Roger . . ."

"I *know* it's low, Bob! But I want the numbers. Now."

"Okay, Roger," I shrugged. "Last time it was 7,500 . . ."

"That was a week ago. What was it before that?"

I told him, tersely, angry at being forced to do so.

Roger digested the figures, drew a long, shuddering breath. "At that rate, Bob, I've got months . . . possibly weeks left. Right?"

I nodded miserably.

He looked at me accusingly. "Have you picked up a copy of *Fit for Life* yet?"

"I've been busy . . ." I began.

"Busy . . . yeah . . ." He didn't finish his sentence. He arose slowly, feebly from his chair and began shuffling down the hall.

Instead of going home for lunch, I stopped at Crown Bookstore and picked up a copy of *Fit for Life*. I carefully skimmed the book before my first patient came in. Though much the author said made sense, I saw nothing in the book that even remotely spoke to AIDS and Roger Cochran. If only the man were on his feet again, I thought, this book would *keep* him well. But, at this point, my task was to *get him well.*

And that I simply did not know how to do.

Mary and the children were back East visiting her mother so I fixed myself a sandwich and carried it to my office. Almost automatically I picked up *Toxemia Explained*. Somehow I was becoming imbued with a strange conviction that somewhere in Tilden's book lay the answer I sought.

For a time I read, my eye catching phrases here and there: "Every so-called disease is built within the mind and body by enervating habits. . . . Nature returns to normal when enervating habits are given up. . . . Using nerve energy in excess of normal production brings on enervation. . . . Perfect health cannot be established until all enervating habits have been eliminated."

Enervation. It seemed to be one of Tilden's key words. I began to look for them and mark them.

"When nerve energy is dissipated from any cause—physical or mental excitement or bad habits—the body becomes enervated. When enervated elimination is hindered, the retention of toxin in the blood causes toxemia. Once established, this accumulation of toxin will continue until nerve energy is restored *by removing the causes. . . .*"

That made good sense.

If the blood is full of toxic waste, the body is sick. The body *must* get rid of that waste, I reasoned, or it will continue to be sick . . . *or sicker* . . . and even die.

I sat bolt upright in my chair.

It isn't virus infection that Roger has. It's toxemia. It's uneliminated poisons!

Roger's body is so full of uneliminated poisons that his overloaded, overworked immune system can no longer handle it. Roger isn't dying of AIDS, I realized. He's dying of *toxemia*: uneliminated waste products in his body!

I could hardly contain myself.

But there was more.

"At first," wrote Tilden, "I believed that enervation

115

must be the general cause of disease; then I decided that simple enervation is not disease, that disease must be due to poison. And that poison, to be the general cause of disease, *must be autogenerated.* What is the cause of that autogeneration? . . .

"It took a long time to develop the thought that a poisoned or injured body, when not overwhelmed by toxemia, would speedily return to normal . . ."

Did that mean, I asked myself, that if by some means Roger could be cleansed of toxemia that he would recover? I jumped up and paced the floor. "Oh, God, let it be so. Let it be so!"

I read on:

"In a few words: *Without toxemia there can be no disease.* I knew," wrote Tilden in words of fire that burned themselves into my brain and spirit, "that the waste product of metabolism was toxic, and that the only reason why we were not poisoned by it was because it was removed from the system as fast as it was produced. Then, I decided, that toxins were retained in the blood *when elimination was hindered.*

"That meant that the cause of elimination hindrances had to be determined. In time I thought out the cause.

"I knew," wrote this man who changed my life and medical practice forever, "that, when we possess normal nerve energy, organic functioning is normal. Then I realized that *enervation* was the hindering cause of improper or imperfect elimination.

"Eureka!" wrote Tilden, "I have found the cause of all disease! *Retention of metabolic waste is the first and only cause of disease!*"

"Eureka!" I shouted with Dr. J. H. Tilden. Unbidden Shakespeare's wisdom immortalized in "Julius

Ceasar" came to mind: "The good that men do live after them . . . so let it be with Tilden."

I wanted to call my wife and give her the news. But with my hand on the telephone, I held back. "Wait, Bob!" I said. "There's yet another step . . . how do you go about cleansing Roger of all that poison in his system? How can you do it and not further weaken—or kill—him?"

I strongly desired to race over to Roger's squalid hotel room and shout the news in his ear. But for the same reason I refrained. I believed with all my heart that I now possessed the knowledge of the cause of Roger's death-dealing AIDS.

But I still lacked one vital link: The way to eliminate all the toxemia from Roger's stricken body.

And the *time* to do it before he became another victim of the dread AIDS that always appears linked to the word *fatal*.

Can I do it?

I finally went to sleep with that question bombarding both my conscious and unconscious mind.

CHAPTER FOURTEEN

I was the first one up and jogging on the San Vicente
median strip the next morning. As I pounded my
usual three miles on the well-packed turf, I reviewed
what I knew must be my procedure. Exhilerated,
both by the stimulating exercise and the prospects of
the new medical frontier I was exploring, I bettered
all my previous times around my track and had showered and was on my way to the hospital thirty minutes earlier than usual.

I parked my car in the hospital parking lot and
checked the dash clock. Still early. *Good*, I thought, *I
can read for a few minutes.* I slid my now-familiar
copy of Tilden's book from my brief case and turned
to a marked section on page 11. Not wanting to miss
a single word, I read aloud, slowly:

"A fast, rest in bed, and the giving-up of enervating
habits, mental and physical, will allow nature to eliminate the accumulated toxin. Then, if enervating
habits are given up, and rational living habits
adopted, *health will come back to stay. This applies
to any so-called disease.*"

I repeated that last sentence several times.

There was a new spring in my step when I entered Surgery.

Two appendectomies later I chanced upon David Cohen in the cafeteria polishing off his usual breakfast. I ordered a large fresh-squeezed orange juice and whole grain toast.

"How's the AIDS patient?" he asked.

"A bit discouraged yesterday," I told him. "But Roger's a tough cookie. He'll fight to the very end . . ."

"To the end?" David asked, a bite halfway to his mouth. "Are you giving up on him?"

"No way, David. No way."

"Oh, say, Bob, last night after you left . . . I stayed a little late . . . a woman came by and dropped off a package for you."

"Oh, who was she?"

"Nice looking lady. Mid-twenties I'd judge. She asked me to see that you got it. I put it on your desk."

I thanked David and promptly forgot the incident.

The waiting room was jammed with patients when I got there, so I actually didn't get to my desk until mid-afternoon. But when I took a brief break and relaxed behind my desk, the first thing I saw was a medium-size, plain manilla envelope. No mailing label. No return address. Just my name hand-printed on the front. Inside was a small paperback book and a note.

Dear Doctor Smith,
Thanks for your kindness to me. Larry has decided to go this route. I'll let you know what happens.

Jennifer

The book was titled, *Fasting Can Save Your Life*,

written by Herbert M. Shelton.

Even though I was extremely busy, the rest of the afternoon went much too slowly to suit me. On the way home I picked up a salad at the deli and prepared to settle down in my study to examine the book.

To my utter amazement, I soon found my now-good friend, Dr. John Tilden mentioned and quoted a number of times in Shelton's book. And I was both pleased and surprised at how much the two writers held in common. "Nothing known to man," Shelton said, "equals the fast as a means of increasing the elimination of waste from the blood and tissues. . . .

"As the fast progresses pent-up secretions or, more properly, retained waste, are thrown out of the body and *the system becomes purified*. Relief of irritations occurs; the body becomes rested. In a vital sense the individual is 'made over.' "

I leaned back in my chair and closed my eyes. "Thank God," I said, "another piece of the puzzle is falling into place."

It was long after midnight when I turned off the light and went to bed. But even in bed, sentence after sentence, even whole paragraphs replayed themselves over in my mind. One that gripped me in particular was in the chapter titled, "Fasting in Acute Disease."

"Instead of fasting being a cure," Shelton wrote, "it is *an essential and integral part of the healing process*."

That jolted me. Then thrilled me.

"When the digestive system is prostrated and all desire for food is cut off, as it is in acute disease, we have an expedient that is as much a part of the remedial process, the process of restoration, and the concomitant prostration of the body as a whole that sends the sick person to bed."

The next sentence, I believed was the key to Roger's return to health . . .

"To be extremely precise, *the fasting process is an actual part of the remedial process that we call disease.*"

Disease: a remedial process! This was a new thought that was to consume my thinking for days.

And fasting an actual part of that *remedial process.*

With all of these new and exciting concepts filling my mind, it's little wonder that I could not sleep.

The next morning, before leaving for the hospital, I phoned Mary. "How's the vacation? And the kids? And you?" I asked all in rapid succession and one breath.

"Wow!" Mary laughed. "You *must* miss us."

"I do miss you," I said, "very, very much. In every way. I love you and wish you were here with me . . . or I with you."

"I love you, too, Bob. All of us are fine . . . spending time resting, reading . . . and just getting caught up on family things. Mother's doing well, so we're having a wonderful time."

She paused at the end of her sentence, but I sensed she was going to say more. I was right. "How's Roger?"

"Actually, Hon, I wanted to discuss him with you . . ."

"Oh? Then he's doing better?"

"No, not really. But, Mary, I now believe I've found the last and final piece of the puzzle . . ."

"That's wonderful. What is it?"

"There's really too much to tell in just a few minutes. But I have a plan . . . actually, it's both a plan and a favor . . ."

"A favor? Of me?"

"Yes, Mary, a big one." I hesitated, trying to remember how I had phrased it during the night. "Well, it's this: I honestly think that we, you and I working together, can save Roger's life."

"I don't understand. How can I help?"

"Mary, Roger needs personal attention . . . he needs us. He needs to stay with us for a while. In our sun room . . ."

She was silent for a moment. "Of course, Bob. But won't we need a nurse as well? I'm willing to do all I can, but . . ."

"I know that, Mary. I knew I could depend upon you. And I will get a nurse for him. I can arrange all of that. But, do you mind if I move him right away?"

"Right away? But I should come home first and take care of things . . . I should . . ."

I broke in. "No, Hon, you shouldn't come home yet. You've got another week with your mother and family. Roger's got to move now. Today."

"Is it really urgent?"

"Yes, I believe it's a matter of life and death . . ."

"But, Bob, who will cook for him? And . . ."

"Mary, that's just it. Nobody will cook for him. He won't be eating. He will be fasting."

After I hung up I chuckled at Mary's response. I could hardly blame her for being puzzled at my new therapy. But no more than I was myself, because, never in my life had I ever heard of a patient, or anybody that I knew, fasting for more than a few hours. Or a day or so at the most.

I made two more calls before leaving for the hospital. Then, satisfied that all was in order, I quickly dressed and let myself out of the house.

All my patients were on time, everything went smoothly, and I left the office promptly at five. Fifteen minutes later I picked up Roger—bag and baggage—and drove him to our home. He protested weakly, "But, Bob, I don't understand. Your home isn't a hospital. And I . . ."

The maid had prepared everything. The sun room bed was made up, the curtains drawn and the late afternoon sun was pouring in. I was pleased at how pleasant and *healing* it looked. I set Roger's suitcase down and seated him near the window.

"And you, my good friend, don't need a hospital. You need a home. Tender, loving care. Lots of fresh air. Sunshine. Rest. I can assure you, you'll get all of that right here."

"But, I still don't understand, Bob. You were so mysterious on the phone this morning. What's this all about?"

I sat down across from Roger. For a moment it was difficult to remember the Roger I had gone to school with, had worked with in Viet Nam. The sagging shoulders, thin, emaciated face and hands. Tired eyes and voice. With an act of will I thought of him as he would be within a few weeks.

"Roger, let me explain . . . I read Diamond's book," I told him. "The man's done a superb job . . . he is doubtless pointing millions of people in the right direction—as far as their eating is concerned . . ."

I paused and let that sink in.

"But right now, it isn't eating you need . . ."

Roger looked up. "I guess not, Bob. I'm not very hungry, if that's what you mean . . ."

"That's partly what I mean," I began.

I shared with him the essence of my discoveries: Tilden's writings. And Shelton's. As I spoke, something of my excitement infected him. He lifted his head and the vestige of a smile came to his lips. His dry humor returned. "So, now you've got me where you want me," he said, "and you're going to starve me to death."

I chuckled. "Right, Roger. I'll get you well in one way or another. And this seemed like the fastest . . ."

"Pun intended?"

We both laughed. And for a moment it was like old times.

"Seriously," I said after we had enjoyed the interlude, "I'm not going to starve you totally. At least not at first."

"Oh? Just partial starvation?"

"That's right. I'll be giving you fruit juice. Several times a day. All fresh squeezed."

Roger seemed to relax visibly. He kicked his shoes off and put his stockinged feet on the hassock. "That sounds good, Bob. So very good . . ."

"And, good buddy," I said, "you're to do nothing. Nothing at all. Except go to the bathroom. Sleep. And lie in the sun. Don't even read for the first few days. What we're going to do is give your body the opportunity it needs to heal itself."

My friend sighed deeply. "Bob, that sounds so good to me. I'm so tired . . . so very tired. Too tired even to thank you properly . . . I'd like to go to bed now. Is that alright?"

"Absolutely. Forget about the thanks. All the thanks Mary and I expect is for you to get well . . . and you *will* do that. I promise."

Roger roused himself momentarily. "But, Mary,

125

this will make a lot of extra work for her . . .
and . . ."

"And, nothing, Roger. The nurse will be here all
day. She'll prepare your juice for you. She'll see to it
that you don't do anything . . . or need anything.
Her name's Ellen. She'll be here in about fifteen minutes . . ."

"By that time I'll be asleep. I can hardly stay
awake."

"Then don't stay awake, Roger. Slide right into
bed. I'll hang your clothes up . . ."

I turned to go, then said, "Roger, I'll pop in several
times during the day. But I won't bother you. I'll
check you over each evening. That's all. Now, *get
well*! That's an order, Doctor!"

He nodded from his bed. His eyes were closed. I
could see his lips moving, but I heard no sound. Before I left the room he was snoring softly.

When Ellen came, I gave her instructions and
showed her to her room. Then I retired to my study
with my two treasures: Tilden and Shelton. However,
this evening I was in bed before nine, and for the first
time in weeks, slept the whole night through.

CHAPTER FIFTEEN

This fasting business was so totally new to me that I found myself feeling like a junior intern. The only time I had ever personally fasted was when I was a teenager. A guest missionary had challenged us to "fast and pray" for missions. Not having a clear understanding of all that was involved, I decided to take him up on it. So I "fasted" or skipped lunch a couple of times. But I was never sure that God heard my prayers, because in anticipation of the "fast," I had eaten a late breakfast which I followed with an early dinner.

Even after reading Shelton's book, I wasn't at all sure what to expect from my patient. I think I half expected Roger to fall over in a faint from weakness. Actually, just the opposite was the case. But not immediately.

I looked in on him the next morning before going to the hospital, but he was sleeping peacefully. At noon I tapped on his door, but he didn't answer, so I didn't look in. Ellen told me he'd taken his fresh fruit juices twice during the morning, then had gone back to bed.

"I've hardly heard a peep out of him," she said.

"I think he was just totally, absolutely exhausted," I told her. "And that's part of what AIDS is all about: exhaustion."

"Exhaustion?" she asked. "I don't understand. Isn't AIDS caused by a virus?"

"Ellen, there are all sorts of theories being bandied about, and that's one of them. Personally, I think AIDS is the result of an abusive lifestyle that has destroyed or nearly destroyed the immune system . . ."

"But, doesn't it work the other way?" she asked. "Doesn't AIDS destroy the immune system?"

"I don't think so, though I know that that's the general theory. Personally I'm of the opinion that AIDS doesn't *attack* either people *or* their immune system. I believe that AIDS develops in people whose lifestyles overburden or break down their immune systems . . ."

She nodded slowly. "That's a new concept to me," she said. "I guess I've got a lot to learn, about AIDS, Doctor."

I nodded. "We've all got a lot to learn about AIDS."

I rapped on Roger's door around six that evening.

"Come in. Come in."

Roger was lying flat in bed. He grinned lopsidedly. "Hi, Doc. Making your rounds?"

"Just checking on my favorite patient. How do you feel? And how have you been doing?"

Roger took a deep breath. "I'm still terribly tired. And I don't feel very well. But, that's nothing new . . ."

"Any special problems?"

"I'm very nauseated. Threw up a couple of times. My head aches. My back hurts something terrible. But I'll live . . ."

"Of course you'll live. Right now it's not the AIDS that's making you sick. It's your body. What's happening to you is something you've probably never heard of before . . ."

"Try me. I've heard of about everything."

"You're going through a *healing* crisis."

Roger laughed without humor. "Here I thought I was sick. And you tell me it's a healing crisis? What's a healing crisis?"

"Your body's working hard to get you well. It's doing it's best to get rid of all the poison you've been storing up for a long time . . ."

Roger gave me a wry smile. "It sounds far out." He shrugged. "But . . ."

"Other than those symptoms, how are you doing?"

Roger made a sweeping motion to include the room. "Bob, this is wonderful. I guess I didn't know how tired I was . . . and how much effort I was expending just to take care of myself. And now all this, including a fulltime nurse. What more could I ask?"

"Are you enjoying the fruit juices?"

"Some of it. I can't drink very much."

"Don't drink any more than you really want. Your body is trying to train you . . . let it do it."

I sat down beside him. "Roger, I'm not going to bother examining you tonight. You need the rest. But, beginning tomorrow evening, I'm going to examine you thoroughly . . . and document every change or improvement. Okay?"

He nodded. "Okay, you call the shots."

"Remember, Roger, this is uncharted ground we're covering. And in the truest sense of the word you're a guinea pig . . ."

"I know. And I feel like a guinea pig. A very sick one."

129

"Sorry about that, Roger. And you might even get sicker. But I believe we're on the right track. And what we're learning might just save a good many lives. So my orders to you are: get well."

Roger moved to get more comfortable, wincing in pain as he did so. "It's my back, Bob. Like I told you, it really hurts."

I made a note of that. "I'll check with you in the morning. So sleep well. Tomorrow, put a 'Do Not Disturb' sign on your door and move outside on the deck for a sun bath. Just a short one. Fifteen minutes front. Same for your back. Then take a luke-warm shower. A brief one. Then get back in bed. Okay?"

"Okay, Doc. I promise."

This kind of therapy was as new to me as it was to Roger. I found myself thinking of prescribing antibiotics, but reminded myself that he didn't need them. He needed only to be left "intelligently alone" to let the body do the work it was best designed to do: to heal itself.

Somewhat disturbed at this new information, I thought, Why hadn't I been doing what I was learning to do now—to *listen* to and obey my own body, and to my patients' bodies? And to teach them the same? I counted the years I had been ministering to sick bodies and wondered how much more good I could have done if I had been doing less drugging and cutting . . .

About two weeks earlier, I had begun trying to treat my patients differently, prescribing fewer drugs, giving fewer shots, and explaining why I was doing what I was doing. Surprisingly, some patients reacted negatively.

"Look, Doc," one crusty patient spoke with considerable agitation, "don't tell me how to run my life. I don't feel well! Just give me something to make me feel better . . ."

"Mister Harris, if you'll be more careful what you eat . . . quit eating all that greasy fried food and . . ."

"I've eaten my fried pork chops all my life. And it's never bothered me. Why should I stop now?"

"I'm trying to tell you that it *is* bothering you. You're eating too much fat. Too much sugar. If you'll ease up on both of them you will start feeling better. Otherwise . . ."

Harris was suddenly angry. "Doctor, I don't tell you how to run your life. And I don't appreciate you trying to run mine for me. I enjoy my life as it is. Eating's about all I've got left. Just leave me alone . . . give me a shot or a prescription. Or something . . . then I'll be okay."

I shrugged and pulled out my prescription pad. "Okay, Mr. Harris . . . get this filled. Tell Janine to schedule you in about two weeks."

Watching Harris hobble away with his cane, I just shook my head. During the two years he'd been my patient, the man had developed diabetes. One of his toes had already turned dark. During his last visit I had suggested the need to remove it and he'd thrown a fit. "I was born with all of my toes," he shouted. "And I'll die with all of my toes. And everything else . . ."

I realized I could do little with the man, other than try to keep him as happy and comfortable as possible.

Another patient, a quite attractive, though very obese young lady, had begged, "Give me some shots to make me lose weight."

"Miss Jenkins, I could give you shots . . . but they really will do you little good. And they can do a lot of harm . . ."

She began crying. "I know I'm eating too much, Doctor. But I can't stop eating. I'm so unhappy. That's why I eat. Then I get fatter and get more unhappy. I think it's a metabolism problem. It's awful. If you'd only give me something to take away my appetite . . . can't you do that?"

Again I tried to explain. "Miss Jenkins, we tested you. And you don't have a metabolism problem. It's . . ."

That's as far as I got when she arose in a huff. "If you won't do it, I'll go to another doctor. My girl friend did and she lost weight . . ."

"I'm sorry, Miss Jenkins," I said. "But going that route could permanently damage your health . . ."

"I don't care if it does. I want to be skinny. *Now*!" She glared at me with tear-reddened eyes. "Doctor, please give me something . . ."

"I'm sorry . . ."

"Then I'm going!" She slammed out of the examining room and was gone. She hadn't returned.

A few others did appreciate my efforts. But not many.

David Cohen remarked about this one day at lunch. "A couple of your patients have come to me," he said. "They told me you refused to treat them. Is that true?"

"Which ones?" I asked, and he named them. I shook my head. "No, David, I didn't refuse to treat any of those patients. But I did refuse to treat them the way they wanted me to treat them. So they got angry and told me they weren't coming back."

He frowned. "Wouldn't it be better to humor them a little? That way you wouldn't lose them . . ."

"Perhaps. But I'm finding it more and more difficult to treat them in ways I know are not in their best interests."

He toyed with his food with his fork. "How is Roger?"

"He's doing about as well as I can expect."

"How's that?"

"He's been complaining of severe back pains and headaches."

"What treatment is he receiving?"

"Rest. Fresh air. Sunshine. Plenty of fluids. Fresh fruit juices . . ."

David raised his eyebrows. "Medication?"

"None . . ."

"None? Do you realize what you're doing, Bob?"

"I think I do."

"Is he responding to your treatment?"

"It's too early to tell . . ."

Neither of us spoke much after that and drove back to the office in silence. It was that afternoon that the letter came. Janine's face was white when she handed it to me. "It's from Jennifer," she said.

"Jennifer? Should I know her?"

"Jennifer Winters. She came in last month. Wanted to talk to you about her friend, Larry . . ."

"Yes, I remember. She thought he might have AIDS. She was the one who sent me the book on fasting. What did she say?"

Janine thrust the letter into my hands. "You read it."

The letter was a single sheet of yellow paper, hand-written. It contained only a few lines . . .

Doctor Smith, Larry died yesterday. He and I read the book I sent you, then he began to fast. Instead of getting better, he just got sicker and sicker. The

end was terrible. He was in an awful lot of pain.
Just thought you'd like to know.

Jennifer

I was stunned. "Can we reach her?"

Janine shook her head. "I don't know how. There
was no return address on her letter. I've checked the
address and phone number she gave me . . . they're
non-existent."

To compound my feelings of failure, when I looked
in on Roger that night, he looked worse than I had
ever seen him. He barely moved or acknowledged my
presence. His skin was cold and clammy, his breathing fast and shallow. The deep, hacking cough he'd
been developing was deeper and more congested. I
caught Ellen's eye and motioned her to follow me
outside.

In the hallway, I asked her, "How has he been doing today?"

She shook her head. "Not good. He hasn't slept
much, and even then he was very restless."

"I'm concerned about that cough?"

"So am I," she said. "He began coughing this
morning. And he's been coughing like you heard him
all afternoon."

"Any other complaints?"

She hesitated. "I don't quite know what to say . . ."

"What do you mean?"

"Well, nothing I can quite put my finger on. It's
just that, well . . . he just seems to be deeply discouraged . . ."

CHAPTER SIXTEEN

After three full days of fasting, Roger appeared no better and I worried that I might be doing him harm by continuing. Before leaving for the hospital in the morning I peeked in. Roger was asleep, so I didn't bother him. At noon when I came home for lunch his "Do Not Disturb" sign was on the door.

Ellen was sitting in the family room reading. She looked up when I entered. "How's our patient?" I asked.

She closed her book and shook her head. "Not good, Doctor. He has refused liquids today for the first time."

"Has he been out of bed?"

"Just to go to the bathroom. A few minutes ago he told me he was going to try to sleep . . ."

"Ellen, let's keep a close check on him. Try to talk to him this afternoon . . . then call me. Okay?"

"Yes, I will, Doctor."

When I went into our cheery little yellow nook room where Mary usually served breakfast, I could see that she was plainly agitated about something. Before sitting down, I kissed her. "Honey, let me know what it is. Okay?"

"Okay," she said and clung to me.

"Is it one of the children?"

"Yes . . . it's Bobby."

"Bobby? Is he acting up in school?"

She shook her head. "No . . . he's in his room now. The nurse sent him home with a note . . ."

"A note? Is he sick?"

"No . . . but it's the same thing about vaccinations again."

"Vaccinations? I thought we'd settled that last week."

She sighed. "So did I, Bob. But, apparently they've got a new nurse . . . or new policy . . . or something. Bobby's the only child who has not taken the shots. Some of his friends are making fun of him. And he's embarrassed . . ."

"I can understand that. But he knows why we're not giving him innoculations, doesn't he?"

She wiped her eyes with the edge of her apron. "I tried to tell him. I think he understands. But, it is difficult for a little boy . . ."

"I know that, Mary. Let's eat, then I'll talk to him."

"And you'll call the school?"

"Better than that. I'll go and talk to the nurse."

Bobby was lying on his bed with his eyes scrunched shut. When I sat down beside him he opened them. "Daddy, the kids are calling me a scardy cat for not getting my shots." His chin quivered and he started to cry.

I put my arms around him. "Bobby, it's okay. I'm going to talk to the nurse before I go back to the office . . ."

"But they keep telling me I'm going to die if I don't get my shots. Is that true, Daddy? Will I die if I don't get shots?"

136

I ran my fingers through his wavy hair. "Of course not. It's they who are likely to get sick. And some of them will."

"But why do they make kids get shots?"

"That's a good question, Bobby. Even the courts can't understand that one. It started a long time ago when some people got the idea that innoculations and vacinations would prevent people from getting sick. Maybe they did. But I don't think so. I been reading that more people get sick and have died from innoculations than the ones who have been protected."

The school nurse, it turned out, thought differently, and tried to force the issue. "Doctor Smith, I'm sorry, but Bobby *must* get his flu shots or he can't come back to school. It's the law." She stood with legs apart and arms crossed as though daring me to refute her statement.

"Miss Troy, please don't try to make it difficult . . ."

"Doctor, I believe it's you who's being difficult. Bobby *must* get his flu shot . . ."

"Miss Troy, do you know how many children die from flu shots each year?"

She shook her head violently. "Don't try that strategy on me, Doctor. It won't work. It's my job to see that *all* children get their shots. No exception."

I sighed. "Miss Troy, are you familiar with California Senate Bill Number 942—Section 1, Chapter 7?" As I spoke I unfolded a piece of paper.

"No," she said. "Should I?"

"Yes, you should, because the bill was passed in 1977 and has not been rescinded. This is how it reads: 'Immunization of a person shall not be required for admission to a school or other institution. . . .' "

I looked up. The nurse was quite obviously upset. "Shall I read the rest of it?"

She shook her head. "No. I've heard of that Bill. But it says the only exemptions that apply are religious. Right?"

"Wrong," I said. "Any parent or guardian responsible for a child simply states in a letter that vaccinations or innoculations are contrary to his beliefs . . . any beliefs. That's all it takes . . ."

"But, I don't understand," the nurse began, "I thought that because you're a doctor you'd . . ." She stopped in confusion, then went on, "Well, anyway, you haven't given me a letter. And until you do . . ."

"Miss Troy, the letter is already in your files. All you had to do was check it out. And if you had you would have saved yourself and me this time . . ."

I started to leave, but turned back. "Miss Troy," I said softly, "I have documentary evidence that vaccinations are dangerous, *very* dangerous, and often fatal." With that, I turned on my heel and left the nurse's office.

The more I read about immunizations, the more convinced I became that I should refuse to vaccinate children, or anybody, who requested it. With Roger lying desperately ill of immune system breakdown, caused, it seemed clear, by drug abuse—of which I believed innoculations were an integral part—I was in no mood to administer even more drugs.

My resistance to innoculations didn't happen overnight. It had never made sense to me that the injection of diseased serum into one's bloodstream could promote health. Even in med school I had questioned the practice. But I had gone along with the AMA accepted practice until last week, when I had been adamant in my refusal to have Bobby innoculated, which resulted in this unneccessary confrontation.

Roger's illness and confirming medical history had proven to be a catalyst to the thought that there might be a connection between drug useage (even legitimate drugs) and the onset of AIDS. Now I was committed to becoming better informed on the subject.

The medical concept of AIDS bothered me. *Why*, I wondered, *has a new epidemic suddenly appeared?* What massive abuse or massive infection could have caused such an outbreak of sicknesses that appear similar? Why is the outbreak more widespread in San Francisco? New York? Los Angeles?

And why, of all places, Haiti? On the surface, it didn't make sense.

I could understand the reasons why the early AIDS victims were thought to have come from the the first three "members" of the AIDS "4-H" Club: homosexuals, heroin abusers and hemophiliacs. I also understood that the greatest density of these three categories of "members" were to be found in the big cities.

But I could not understand the rationale for the fourth member of the group: Haitians. The first three had two things in common: drugs and hypodermic needles; both of which included the possibility of mixing or intermingling one's body fluids with those of another *via the needle*. All three of these entities also had a record of drug useage, either legal or otherwise. And it was a fact that drug useage resulted in immuosuppression.

But why the Haitians?

Haiti, I realized, was the poorest country in the Western hemisphere, with a current average income of $300. I asked, *Does poverty cause AIDS?* If such were the case, then the millions of poverty-stricken Americans would be a hot-bed of AIDS, which I knew was not so. And Haitians, as far as I knew, were not known for drug abuse. Or, were they?

As I pondered this question, the answer came: yes and no.

No, the Haitians were not known for heroin abuse. But, yes, they did have a history of *legal* drug useage.

The Haitians' poverty could not, in and of itself, breed AIDS. But it was a fact that the Haitians' poverty does result in disease: endemic diseases such as tuberculosis, typhoid fever, bacterial and protozoal dysenteries, malaria, widespread malnutrition, and yaws (an infectious disease caused by bacteria similar to the bacteria that causes syphilis).

To combat Haiti's disease problem, I learned, most, if not all Haitians are *regularly* and routinely treated with immune-suppressing drugs: long-acting penicillin therapy for yaws and innoculations or vaccinations for tuberculosis and typhoid fever. The consistent, and longterm use of those drugs amounted to drug abuse; abuse that was cumulative.

Ergo: *immune response suppression.*

The very symptom presently diagnosed as AIDS.

By projection, drug abuse results in the crippling of the immune system. Crippling of the immune system results in AIDS.

Putting two and two together equalled my answer.

Haiti's problem was *drug abuse!*

It mattered not a whit that the drug abuse was legal. The end result was exactly the same.

My concern was further heightened and my resistance to innoculations strengthened by an article I read describing the dilemma faced by our national lawmakers in their implementation of the National Childhood Vaccine Injury Act of 1986.

"Congress has been unable to agree on a method to fund the program," the report read, "which is *designed to compensate families of children who are injured or die as a result of vaccinations for diptheria, pertussis, rubella, polio and other illnesses*" ("INSIGHT," March 30, 1987).

Suddenly the whole AIDS picture began coming into sharper focus. Americans routinely innoculate their tiny babies (some of them only a few days or weeks old) with disease-producing "serums" manufactured from repulsive pustules and animal urine. They vaccinate or innoculate these infants not just once, but twice or more.

Followed by immune-suppressing x-rays by dentists and medical doctors, parents' administration of numerous over-the-counter drugs, average poor nutrition, more injections (for a variety of problems, real and suspected) throughout their childhood, our infants' original DPT shots start the ball rolling for the early beginning for the drug-induced suppression of our childrens' immune systems.

After that beginning, it's merely a matter of time until the heroic efforts of abused immune response systems falter (result: chronic illness) and begin to fail (result: numerous terminal degenerative diseases such as cancer, heart disease, arthritis, osteoporosis and AIDS).

Could their progress be halted?

I hoped so.

For 40,000 American AIDS victims, including my friend Roger Cochran, the time had come.

CHAPTER SEVENTEEN

Mary was shaking me. "Wake up, Bob. Wake up!" she whispered.

"Uh, what?"

"Wake up. Somebody's knocking on our door."

"Our door?" I sat up. As I did I became aware of the soft tapping. "Who's there?" I shouted.

"It's me. Ellen. Come quick."

"Why? What's the matter?"

"It's Roger," her voice was muffled through the door. "I think something's wrong . . . hurry. Please hurry."

The face of my illuminated clock read eleven-thirty. We'd been in bed less than an hour. I shook my head to clear away the cobwebs. "Be right there." I struggled into my robe.

Ellen's face was strained in the dim hall light. "Tell me what happened," I said as we moved down the hall.

"I was asleep in the adjoining room. And Roger's groans woke me." She pulled her dressing gown closer and shivered. "Sounded like he was in terrible pain . . ."

"Did you go into his room?"

"Yes . . . he was lying on his side, clutching his stomach with both hands. And . . . and groaning."

By then we were downstairs and I could hear Roger's moaning. I could see light under the door. I entered without knocking. Roger was sitting up in bed, rocking back and forth, holding his head with both hands. His eyes were closed. If he heard us enter he gave no indication. As he rocked, those terrible groans seemed to be forced from deep within him.

I gripped one of his shoulders. "Roger. Roger!"

He opened his eyes wide and I saw they were sunken and filled with pain. He focussed on me and at first I wasn't sure that he knew me.

"Roger . . ."

"Hi, Bob," he mumbled thickly. "This is awful. My head. My stomach. My legs and back. I hurt all over. Oh, God, it hurts!"

He looked so miserable I wished I could do something.

Roger must have read my mind. "I don't think I can stand much of this . . ." He groaned and clutched his back. "Can you give me something for this, Bob . . . some codeine, Excedrin? Or anything? Please."

For one long moment I wavered. Was it worth it? Was all this discomfort doing anything positive for Roger. Anything at all? Maybe I could, or should, give him something to ease the pain. Or put him in the hospital . . .

Then I remembered how he looked when he came to me. Orthodox medicine had done all it could do for Roger, which had amounted to exactly nothing. They had given up on him and had consigned him to an early grave. Even Roger himself had all but given up.

Roger and orthodox medicine had tried the drug route and it had failed. It had failed because drugs had been the cause of his problem in the first place. And more drugs had only exacerbated the problem they had caused. In that one crystal clear moment, I knew that hospitals . . . orthodox medicine . . . drugging *were not* the answer for Roger.

They could not bring life and health back to my friend.

For nearly a week, now, Roger had been free of drugs of all kinds. He had not so much as seen or touched even an aspirin. He had not tasted anything but pure, fresh fruit juice and fresh, pure water. Nothing else had gone into his body . . .

He may not have evidenced measureable progress during that week. But he had not regressed.

That meant that even though Roger had shown no overt signs of improvement, the mere fact that he had not lost ground was in itself improvement!

Suddenly I knew: If I weakened now, gave up, returned Roger to the hospital and to the ministrations of orthodox medicine, it would be the beginning of the end. And we would never reach this place again. All of this came to me in that millisecond when Roger had begged for relief.

I shook my head. "No, Roger. No. No drugs."

"Please," he begged. "I can't stand this . . ."

My moment of weakness had passed. I grabbed Roger by the arm and pulled him to a seating position. Over my shoulder I spoke to Ellen. "Go run the tub full of warm water. We'll let Roger soak a while. That should help."

She left without a word. Moments later I heard water running. Roger was so weak that we had to half carry him into the bathroom and help him into the tub. By the time we got him into the tub all three of us were perspiring. Ellen and I from the unaccustomed exertion. Roger from the exertion and pain.

When Roger felt the warm water closing over him, he groaned, whether in pain or relief I wasn't sure, then sank down in the tub and closed his eyes. Ellen and I were panting. She sat on the bath stool; I leaned against the wall. We watched him without saying a word.

After a while he relaxed somewhat and stretched out full length. A grin creased his mouth. "Sorry, old buddy . . ."

"That's alright. How are you feeling now?"

"Better, I think . . ."

"Don't talk. Just relax."

I motioned to Ellen, "I'll handle him now. Thanks for your help. Just go on back to bed. Try to get some sleep. Okay?"

She nodded gratefully. "I'll be available if you need me."

Roger closed his eyes and visibly relaxed some more. I felt the temperature, then warmed up the water. For a while the only sounds were Roger's somewhat labored breathing and the drip of water into the tub.

Finally Roger stirred, opened his eyes and looked up. "Oh. Oh . . . I guess I went to sleep." He stretched his arms and flexed his knees.

"Feeling better?"

His grin was less strained. "Better, I think. Really, *much* better." He sat up and twisted his shoulders and back. "Yes . . . much, much better."

He looked up. "Bob, I've never felt anything quite like this before. It seemed that all my muscles just knotted up—all over my body—and I couldn't get them to let go. It was terribly painful."

"You say it's never happened like this before?"

He shook his head. "No. Not really. A few times I've gotten cramps, sort of charlie horses, but not like this." He prodded his back and sides with his fingers. "It's a lot better now. The knots have gone away." He sighed deeply. "I think I can rest now, and maybe sleep."

I squeezed his wet shoulder. "Good, Roger. I'll help you get comfortable."

Mary snuggled close to me when I got back in bed, but made no sound. My mind was in a whirl. *I didn't drug him*, I thought, *I didn't drug him. And he got through this crisis without it*! When I finally slept I dreamed that Roger and I were standing back to back, fighting off a bunch of drunk sailors in a Saigon bar.

Though he fasted for two more weeks, from that night on, Roger began showing definite signs of improvement. The signs were minute, but definitive.

David Cohen shook his head when I told him. "Don't get too optomistic, Bob. It's probably just a temporary remission. That happens, you know."

"I know about remissions, David. And I agree, it's possible that this *could be* nothing but temporary. But I don't think so."

"Forgive me for being pessimistic," David went on, "but I've seen cancer do that. And AIDS is like a cancer in several respects. It's tricky. When a temporary or false remission takes place, the patient suddenly feels good for a day or two. Or a week. Maybe a month. Then all at once he takes a nosedive. And that's it. The end."

"I agree. I've seen remissions like that, too. But, not this one. This one is different . . ."

"Different?" David raised his eyebrows. "In what way?"

"There's a freshness about Roger's skin. It seems to have lost its pasty color and quality. His eyes have a new sparkle to them . . ."

"Has he gained any weight?"

"No. He's still losing weight. He's down to less than 140."

I expected David's response. "Bob, be reasonable. If your patient *seems* to be feeling better, and *seems* to be looking better . . . those are subjective measurements. And they don't count. You're a doctor, you know that."

"You're right, David. But there's more."

"More?"

"Right. I haven't forgotten the objective tests."

"Oh . . . such as?"

"For one thing, Roger's white blood cell count is up. And, another thing, his T4/T8 ratio is improving . . ."

"What?" The tone of David's voice was incredulous. "Are you *sure*? I've never heard of that before, not in any AIDS patient."

I nodded. "Nor have I. But I've checked and rechecked. I'm sure I'm right. It's definite: The white cell count has increased about five percent. And his total number of lymphocytes has risen significantly . . ."

We both knew that a body's T4/T8 lymphocyte ratio is often considered to be the barometer of the immune system. And that without adequate T4 helper cells to prod the immune system into battle, or sufficient T8 suppressor cells to tell the immune system to lay down its arms when the fight is finished, the whole system would be out of commission.

David gave a low whistle. "Bob, that *is* a good sign. A very good sign."

"I know. It means Roger's immune system is no longer dead or dormant. That it's beginning to function again!" I had been quietly elated over this fact and hadn't shared my secret with anyone until this moment. None of the literature I had read had even hinted that any experimental drugs had been able to reverse a patient's immune system dysfunction.

"Have you told Roger?"

"No. You're the very first to hear . . ."

I should have cautioned David to keep the news to himself. But he didn't.

CHAPTER EIGHTEEN

I did my best to play down the "AIDS doctor" bit. After all, the only thing I'd done had been to provide Roger with a quiet, stress-free environment and put him on a voluntary fast. On the other hand, *I had* done something that was very significant: I had withheld drugs.

The response of my colleagues to whatever it was they perceived that I had done, ran the gamut.

Dan Halley slid his tray next to mine. "Congratulations."

"What for?" I was non commital.

"For bringing about such a positive remission in your AIDS patient"

I didn't respond. He stirred his coffee. "Do you know of any other AIDS patient whose immune system has ceased to regress?"

"No, Dan, I don't," I said. "But, then, I don't know any other AIDS patients. Correction, I knew *of* another one . . ."

Dan raised his eyebrows. "You knew *of* another? What happened to him?"

"He died."

"Oh. I'm sorry. But, I guarantee that you'll soon be knowing other AIDS patients."

"I don't think so, Dan. One is enough. It takes a lot of time to work with a person with AIDS."

"I know. But the word will get around. You'll be getting all sorts of applicants."

True to form, Tom Holmes was cynical in his attitude. But he said much less than I anticipated. He fixed me with his piercing blue eyes. "So you took an AIDS patient into your home? Don't you know there are hospices for people like that?"

I knew Holmes' passing comment didn't require an answer, so I just shrugged and said nothing.

The grapevine in a hospital is very active, and the word got around that I had housed an AIDS patient in my home. Within the next few days most of the doctors and some of the nurses stopped me to make a comment or ask a question. This sudden attention made me quite uncomfortable. Though Roger's condition evidently was improving daily, I knew it was far too soon to be making any predictions.

So with Mary I was cautiously optimistic.

And with Roger I was clinically optimistic. "The blood lesions on your feet and legs are getting smaller," I observed one day. "That's a good sign . . ."

He grinned happily. "I know. I've been watching them. Something else, I don't have those awful pains in my muscles and joints like I had for so long. What do you think? Do we have it licked?"

I shook my head. "I don't know. But let's not be too hasty. Let's just say your condition is improving . . ."

"Immensely?" he added.

"Okay," I admitted, "let's add *immensely*."

I checked my chart. "Do you realize how long you've been fasting?"

Without hesitation he said, "Twenty four days today."

Ellen said, "He's sleeping better now. He no longer has such terrible breath. And even though he's been fasting for so long, he actually seems stronger than when he started."

"Are you hungry?"

Roger shook his head. "Not really. The smell of food during meal preparations appeals to me. But, no, actually I haven't been hungry at all."

Physically Roger looked quite skeletal and resembled some pictures I'd seen of starving people. But, paradoxically, his previously baggy skin was beginning to tighten and his muscle tone was improving. And, as a result of his daily sun baths, his skin was taking on a healthy brown tone.

I asked Ellen. "How much did Roger weigh this morning?"

"One hundred thirty five."

"How much has he lost since beginning to fast?"

"We didn't weigh him until he'd been fasting for a couple of days. But since I've been weighing him, Roger has lost a total of nine pounds. Actually, he didn't have much left to lose . . ."

"Not when his normal weight is around two hundred," I said.

However, I had to admit that my patient was giving me much to feel optimistic about, especially as I noted a marked decrease in the size of the Kaposi's sarcoma blood lesions on his feet and legs. Roger's chest congestion was clearing as well, and I rarely heard him coughing at night.

As I watched Roger stand and walk with less discomfort, I allowed myself the luxury of thinking, *Maybe the remission is genuine. Maybe he will recover.* The thought was strengthened one day as I was driving home for lunch and saw Roger, with Ellen beside him holding his arm, out walking a block or so from home.

I slowed down and honked. They both waved and Roger shouted, "This feels great!"

Ellen said nothing, but she did smile happily.

I mentioned the incident to Mary. She put on her Mona Lisa face and remarked, "Hadn't you noticed?"

"Noticed what?"

"How Roger and Ellen look at each other?"

"Well, yes, he does depend upon her a great deal. And she's an excellent nurse . . . quite a pretty one, at that," I added.

"Pretty *and* single?"

"And single. Say, Mary, you're right. Something just might be developing between them. That would be wonderful."

To myself I thought, *Couldn't it be, that the quite apparent affection Roger and Ellen are beginning to show for each other also has something to do with his physical improvement?"*

Mary voiced my thoughts. "Bob, I truly believe that Roger's healing, if we can call it that, has at least *something* to do with the personal attention Ellen is giving him. As as well as what I perceive to be her love. Don't you?"

I took a generous bite of my sandwich and shook my head. "You may be right about that? We know that a person's emotional state—feelings of fear or rejection . . . frustration . . . anger, especially unresolved anger . . . unforgiveness, either toward himself or toward another—all of these things are able to effect physiological and chemical changes within one's body . . ."

Mary was idly tracing a pattern on the tablecloth with her finger. She nodded. "And didn't you tell me that Roger was devastated when his wife left him?"

"Yes. It happened while he was in Viet Nam. Roger was pretty bitter about it . . . started hitting the bottle pretty heavily. And got into drugs."

"Then you think that his emotional state, *along with* his chemical addiction might have been at least partially responsible for his physical degeneration?"

"Absolutely, Mary. Absolutely."

My wife looked up and beamed her lovely, heart-stopping smile upon me. "Then, if Roger's emotional state helped to bring about his physical degeneration, the reversal of those emotions *could* effect positive changes? In his body as well as his mind?"

"You're right again, Mary . . ."

We heard the front door open and heard Ellen's tinkling laughter, followed by Roger's deep bass chuckle.

Mary smiled. "Aren't those 'healing-in-progress' noises?"

I squeezed her hand. "Leave it to a woman . . ."

That afternoon, Glenda Horowitz, an arthritis patient, had a book in her hand when she came into the Treatment Room. "What are you reading, Glenda?"

She handed it to me. Written by someone named Paavo O. Airola, a man I'd never heard of, the book was titled, *There Is a Cure for Arthritis*. I noticed that the author was not a medical doctor and was about to hand the book back when I saw that the

Foreward was written by an M.D.

My eye caught, "Bacteria or virus are not primary causes of disease; they are only symptomatic factors. . . . Chemical drugs can, at their best, serve only for the temporary relief of symptoms. Prolonged use of drugs will *always* damage the biological milieu. . . ."

I looked up. Glenda was regarding me intently. I indicated the book. "Have you read this?"

"Yes, I have," she answered me steadily. "And I liked what I read . . . do you?"

"I don't know yet," I answered cautiously.

My eyes jumped to the last paragraphs of the Foreward and caught the words, "Where the damage effected by the prolonged therapy with chemical drugs and corticosteroids is so extensive that it had caused the glandular atrophy and the impairment in the body's own healing mechanism, or where there are extensive degenerative changes in the joints, then even biological medicine will be but of little help.

"Nevertheless, after reading this book, one must draw the conclusion that every passing year, that conventional medicine, wrapped in *prejudicial thinking*, is unwilling to change its attitude and thinking pattern and ignores the existence of biological medicine, a countless number of people will be subjected to needless and prolonged suffering."

I started to hand the book back to Glenda, then changed my mind and quickly let the pages flip through my fingers. Two headings caught my eye: "Therapeutic Fasting," and "The Vital Role of Nutrition."

During this minute or so, Glenda hadn't uttered a word. I closed the book and handed it to her. "Why did you bring the book?" I asked her.

Though she was nervous, she held my eye. "I found it in B. Dalton Booksellers . . . the drugs you were giving me weren't helping. So I . . . I bought the book. Took it home and read it." She held out her stiff fingers. The joints were red and swollen. "Doctor Smith, I'm only 37. I'm too young to be getting crippled with arthritis. After I read that book I began to hope that there might be a chance . . ."

She faltered and stopped.

"A chance, Glenda?" I asked softly. "A chance for what?"

"A chance that you might . . . you might read the book. And maybe you'd . . . you'd treat me like the book says . . ."

I smiled. "You mean, put you on a fast?"

"Yes, Doctor. I'm afraid to fast by myself. I don't know if I could do it. And . . . and, well, I'm afraid to try it . . . for fear that it wouldn't work. Do you understand?"

"Of course, Glenda. Of course."

In the next few seconds I mentally reviewed this woman's problem. For months I had been giving Glenda drugs for her arthritis, all to no avail, except to dull her pain for brief periods of time. I knew her prognosis wasn't good, that all I could do for her—or any doctor I knew—would be to give her different and possibly stronger drugs to ease her discomfort. But I had to admit that I knew of no way to halt the course of her disease.

Wasn't it possible, the thought came, *that fasting could do something positive for her*? If fasting could do something for a condition as serious—as *fatal*, according to the statistics—as AIDS, then couldn't it be possible, that fasting could change the course of other diseases?

I took a deep breath. "Glenda, did the bookstore have other copies of this book?"

"They did have," she said. "But, why don't you take mine and read it? I can pick it up in a few days."

"Alright, I'll borrow your book. And I promise to read it."

"Will you then at least consider putting me on a fast?"

I looked at the young woman's reddened fingers. *How could a fast hurt her?* I thought. *Why not?* I asked myself.

I stuffed the book into the pocket of my smock. "Glenda, give me a few days to think about it . . . read this book, do some more research. Then I'll call you. Okay?"

The gratitude in Glenda's warm, hopeful smile shamed me. *How can I refuse anything that could possibly help her?* I thought. In my heart I knew that I would not refuse her request. But, along with my strong desire to help Glenda was the fear that I could be wrong and that I might be extending to her a false hope.

Nevertheless, on the way home that evening, I stopped at B. Dalton's Bookstore and purchased three more copies of Airola's book, along with a couple other ones that caught my eye. That evening I handed Ellen, Roger and Mary a copy of Airola's book. "Please read it," I said, "and tell me what you think."

After dinner I retired to my study and, felt-tipped marker in hand, I read every page of Airola's remarkable book.

CHAPTER NINETEEN

"This book is written with the sole aim of bringing good news . . . to millions of arthritis sufferers and freeing them from their hopelessness and desperation," wrote Airola.

I pricked up my ears.

"My happy message to them," Airola went on, "is that they should not despair. Biological medicine has an answer to their problems."

Airola defined biological medicine as the natural method(s) of treating *all manner* of illness and disease. *Including AIDS?* I wondered.

"Since the average practitioner of orthodox medicine does not have a clear understanding of the basic causative principles involved in arthritis," I read, "his treatments and remedies are understandably symptomatic—that is, *he is not treating the disease but the isolated symptoms of the disease.*"

To my wide open mind, practically everything Airola was saying spoke as much to AIDS or any other degenerative disease as it did to arthritis.

". . . arthritis is a systemic disease which *affects the whole body.* (*So does AIDS!* I was thinking.)

Therefore, the only measures that can be successful in correcting the disease, bringing it under control, and accomplishing a lasting cure, must be ones directed at correcting its underlying causes. . . ."

Including AIDS! I agreed.

"This can only be accomplished by treatments which help to overcome the systemic disturbances, normalize the metabolic processes, and help *restore all normal functions* of the vital organs and glands. . . ."

I became aware that I was perched on the edge of my chair, gripping the book with both hands. I felt like shouting "Eureka! I have found it!" to the world.

"While drugs and injections may relieve pain and modify symptoms," I read on, "*they do not go to the bottom of the problem*, they do not eliminate the underlying causes, nor do they correct the systemic disturbances. What is even worse, these conventional remedies, being suppressive in nature and having undesirable toxic side effects, interfere with the normal bodily processes, and actually inhibit restorative and healing efforts of the body. *Eventually they cause more damage than good* and lead to a complete invalidism. . . ."

I laid the book aside and began pacing my office like a caged lion. "Oh, God," I spoke aloud, "why haven't I seen this before?"

My study clock struck eleven o'clock, but I ignored it. I knew Mary would be waiting up for me. But I couldn't leave my office yet. There was more, so very much more to read, to learn, to share.

I picked up the book again.

"It must be emphatically stated that drugs do not possess curative powers. The cure is always brought about by the body itself, and the most that a wise doctor can ever do is assist the body's own healing forces."

And how, I asked myself, *does that wise doctor assist the patient's body to utilize it's own healing forces?*

In that moment of discovery, I knew as well as I knew my own name, that the healing philosophy that Airola was espousing was not earmarked for arthritis alone. Airola was speaking of basic principles that applied to disease in general. All kinds of diseases.

And though Airola did not speak of AIDS by name, I knew in my heart that he was speaking of AIDS as much as he was speaking of arthritis: both the cause and the cure.

He spoke of "systemic disease" that affected the whole body. *AIDS definitely affected the whole body.*

Airola wrote of disease's "underlying problem." Furthermore, he spoke of *discovering* the underlying cause of arthritis, and when he had found it, he had been able to effect a cure, a return to wellness.

Likewise, I believed that I had discovered the underlying cause of AIDS: abusive life style. A life style that included, but was not limited to chemical abuse, physical abuse, sexual abuse, emotional abuse (fear, anger, hatred, unforgiveness and so on), and/or a combination of some or all kinds of abuse.

Furthermore, Airola declared, that when the underlying causes were removed, and correct biological medicine was employed (*Or*, I substituted, *health-giving life principles instituted*), that the body would then, through the activation of it's own inherent healing abilities, restore health and well being to the erstwhile diseased and suffering body.

Somewhere in the back of my head I heard the clock strike midnight, but I could not stop now. I had to go on.

I had to learn the nature of Airola's biological medicine. I must not stop until I discovered the methods he employed. I felt myself gripped by a driving sense of urgency.

"Oh, God," I whispered into my darkened office, "I must learn how to do it . . . how to rescue AIDS victims . . . and all other kinds of victims . . . I must learn how to reach all of them, all those trusting victims that orthodox medicine has doomed to a living death of drug dependence . . ."

My face was wet with tears, but I was unaware of it. "I must teach them how to infuse themselves with this dynamic wellness that is their birthright . . . I must. I must!"

Suddenly I was aware that someone else was in the room. Mary had come in so quietly that I had not noticed. She slipped her arm around my shoulders and whispered, "You will, Bob. You will."

At noon the next day I was met at the door by Roger and Ellen, their faces aglow. "Where did you get that book?" Roger asked.

For a moment I forgot that I had given each of them a copy of Airola's book. "Book?" I asked. "Which book?"

Roger was impatient. "The book you gave us last night. You know, Airola's book, *There Is a Cure for Arthritis*. That book."

I was startled by his vehemence. "Oh. Why? Did you like it?"

"Like it? Bob, it's a great book. Wonderful! In fact, I wish I'd read Airola's book years ago. There's only one thing I'd like to see changed . . ."

"What's that?"

"Well, the author speaks mainly to arthritis. But he's actually talking about principles that should apply to all diseases. Not just arthritis."

"That's right, Doctor Bob," Ellen added shyly. "It's a very helpful book. I liked it a lot. As a nurse it will help me to be much more effective in my work."

"For instance?" I directed my question to Ellen.

"Well, for one thing, for the first time I began to fully understand the principles behind fasting. And I realized what you were trying to accomplish by fasting Roger."

I smiled. "Apparently we're on the right track, aren't we?"

Roger grinned and straightened his shoulders. "That's right, Bob. And I'm grateful. Do you realize this is my *thirty-fifth* day of fasting? With nothing but fresh-squeezed fruit juices and water?"

"Thirty five days?" I said. "Seems like three years to me."

Roger nodded. "In a way it does to me, too. But, Bob, do you personally know anyone who has fasted thirty five days?"

"No, not personally. Roger, you're looking very good. How do you feel?"

"Better than I thought I'd feel, subsisting on just fruit juice and water. And," he reminded, "don't forget, *no drugs* of any kind."

"Right. No drugs," I agreed. "It must be some sort of a record . . ."

"You bet it is. Anyway, to answer you, I feel okay. Weak. Low energy level. But no pain. The pain's all gone. That's the best thing. I've lived with pain for so long . . . anyway, I've got something to show you. Just take a look at this."

He slipped off his sandals and showed me the bottom of his feet. "The blood lesions . . . the Kaposi's sarcoma . . . all gone from my feet. Completely gone. My legs, too. Not a sign."

I rolled my chair closer and ran my fingers over the new, smooth flesh of Roger's feet and legs. There was no sign of a bruise or lesion.

"Roger, that's fantastic! Now *that's* some sort of a medical mile post! That's absolutely wonderful! Any other good news?"

He nodded. "Of course. There's more. I checked my blood pressure today and it's normal . . . for the first time in years it's normal!"

"Normal? Even a week ago it was elevated."

"But not today. And like I said, the pains . . . those terrible pains in my back . . . and my legs . . . they're gone. Bob, I . . ." He started to say more, but choked up with emotion. Ellen reached for his hand and gripped his fingers in her own.

"I think what he wants to say, Doctor, is that . . . that, well . . . he told me this morning, that for the first time he actually thinks he's going to be well again."

I noticed the cheeks of both of them were wet with tears.

About a week later Glenda called. "I'm sorry, Doctor," she began, "but I just couldn't wait any longer. What did you think of Airola's book."

Cautiously I said, "Glenda, I think it holds great promise."

"Then you'll supervise a fast for me?"

"I'm sorry, Glenda," I said, and even over the telephone I could sense her disappointment, "but I'm not equipped to do that for you . . ."

"Oh . . . but I thought . . ."

"Don't give up, though," I said, "I didn't say you shouldn't fast for your arthritis. I think you should. I just told you that I am not equipped to do it myself. And I think if you're going to fast for a period of time you should be supervised."

"But, I don't know anybody . . . or any place . . ."

"I can suggest two places," I told her, "places where trained personnel are able to care for you in ways that I could not . . . and I'll be glad to . . ."

"To put me in touch with them?" Glenda broke in excitedly.

I chuckled. "That's exactly what I was going to tell you. Come in tomorrow and Janine will give you the addresses. You can contact them yourself. Okay?"

"Oh, thank you, Doctor. Thank you."

"I have one request to make."

"Whatever you ask," she said.

"Just keep me informed, please. Keep good notes . . ."

"Keep good notes? But, why?"

"Because I want to be able to recommend places where other patients can go to find relief. From arthritis. And from other problems . . . okay?"

I sensed her relax. "Doctor Smith, I'll be glad to do that for you . . . and for those other patients."

Those other patients just might be AIDS patients, I said to myself.

Even though Roger had shown so much progress, we both agreed that he should not break his fast yet. I realized we were feeling our way through what was to us an uncharted wilderness, but we didn't want to make any mistakes.

"I feel better than I've felt in years," Roger told me on his thirty-fifth day of abstinence from anything except fresh fruit juices. "And I'm sleeping better. In fact, I need only about six or seven hours of sleep a night. That's less sleep that I've ever done without . . ."

I chuckled. "Not I, Roger. I remember Viet Nam. Some of those nights were only two or three hours long?"

He laughed. "I remember those, too. But I mean *normal* time sleep. Viet Nam was different."

Roger was in my office examination room, stripped to his undershorts. "I know I look like a skeleton," he said, half selfconsciously, "and I *am* a little weak. But I don't get as tired as I thought I would . . ."

When he stepped onto the scales it read: 135.

I thought a moment. "Roger, I think it's time to consider taking you off your fast. What do you think?"

He answered slowly. "I suppose so. But I'm not hungry."

"I remember you telling me that. But I think we should begin building up your weight. We'll do it carefully. Feed you nothing but fresh fruits and vegetables. Small quantities at first. Then gradually increase them . . ."

He didn't answer immediately. "I feel so good, Bob, I'm almost fearful of eating. Sounds funny, I guess."

"I think I understand. But I really think it's time."

He nodded. "I do, too." He took a deep breath. "Yes, Bob, I agree. So . . . let's begin."

"Tomorrow morning?" I asked.

"Tomorrow morning." Roger gave me a bear hug. I couldn't help but notice how much stronger he was than when he first walked into my office six months ago.

CHAPTER TWENTY

"AIDS is being heralded as the worst epidemic in the history of mankind," David was telling me. Our last patient had gone home and we were relaxing in my office.

"I know," I told him.

"Do you think it's true?"

I shook my head. "No, I don't. Frankly, I think that's just some more media hype . . ."

"It's bad, though, Bob. You've got to admit that."

"Sure it's bad. Anytime anyone dies before his time it's bad. But bad is a relative term."

"What do you mean?"

"Well, for one thing, how many deaths do you know of that have been blamed on AIDS?" I asked.

David thought for a moment. "The latest figures say about 20,000, give or take a few."

"In how long a period of time?"

"Since 1981."

"Okay, that's between three and four thousand deaths a year connected with AIDS. Do you agree?"

"Sure. But what are you getting at?"

"How many people die of strokes every year?"

David answered immediately. "Close to 350,000."

"And cancer?"

"Approaching half a million a year."

"Do we consider strokes and cancer as being epidemic?"

David shook his head. "I see what you're getting at. But aren't we seeing a constant increase of AIDS patients?"

"Without a doubt. But we're also seeing an increase in the number of deaths from all these other diseases too."

"Okay," David said, "but I hear and read all the time that AIDS is probably one of the worst plagues ever to hit mankind."

Without a word I pulled a book from my shelf and opened it to a marked page. "You know who Dr. Roy Walford is, don't you?"

David nodded. "Sure. He's Professor of Pathology at UCLA School of Medicine."

"Right. And he's held that post since 1966. He's a man you can trust. Right?"

David agreed.

"Okay, listen to what Walford says about plagues. He says, 'Arteriosclerotic heart disease is the greatest epidemic mankind has ever faced, carrying off a larger percentage of the population than the Black Death in the Middle Ages.' "

I held the place with my finger and closed the book. "If we're really talking about plagues . . . something that's running rampant, out of control, I think we'd define something like arteriosclerotic heart disease a plague. A genuine plague."

"But most heart disease can be prevented."

I smiled. "Of course most heart disease can be prevented. And in the opinion of many researchers, even most cancer can be prevented . . ."

"Who, for instance?" he challenged me.

I shrugged and handed him Dr. Walford's book. "Walford says, on page 125, that '80 to 90 percent of cancers are due to environmental factors.' And of those environmental factors, he says diet is the most important."

I took a deep breath. "David, you know that Kaposi's sarcoma is considered to be a type of cancer. It's also one of the so called opportunistic diseases that are said to 'attack' AIDS victims . . ." I paused and David nodded his agreement.

"This means to me that if a high percentage of cancers are caused by environmental factors, AIDS could be included. And if that's so, that means it's not only possible to prevent AIDS, but that *it's also possible to reverse the course of the disease.*"

Driving home that night I replayed my conversation with David. Though I really believed that AIDS was *caused* and not just *caught*, and that AIDS was the effect and not the cause of the immune system breakdown, I had to admit that I didn't actually know how this came about.

To date I had treated only one AIDS patient. One treatment: one recovery, which equalled 100%. Not bad. However, now I had to face the inevitable question: Can I do it again?

I would like to think that the answer was yes.

But I knew it was not possible to give an unqualified yes until I could state an unequivocal cause (or causes) for the immune system breakdown which resulted in the diagnosis of AIDS. In Roger's case we had determined that drug abuse—"legal" drug abuse at that—was probably the most obvious *immediate* cause.

Massive evidence seemed to point to homosexuality *and* the resultant homosexual lifestyle as being the basic cause for the highest percentage of AIDS victims. The "resultant lifestyle" being defined as the stereotypical projected upon those who had adopted a homosexual preference. Into this stereotypical lifestyle mode, non-homosexuals defined and "dumped" such items as chemical addiction (especially needle-injected drugs), including alcohol addiction, promiscuity, emotional instability, plus numerous excesses of every kind.

Some researchers claimed that male semen was the culprit, and that when injected other than in the vagina, it somehow had an extreme negative effect, resulting in all sorts of problems. This I found difficult to believe.

As I sought out, considered and evaluated all the hypotheses and theories, I rejected first one, then another, and soon found myself left with only one or two.

One of these was articulated very well by Dr. Arnold Fox, author of the *Beverly Hills Medical Diet* and other books, in a magazine article titled "Stress and Your Immune System" (LET'S LIVE, January 1987).

Discussing the subject of stress, Dr. Fox asked, "Can your *thoughts* really weaken your immune system?"

"Yes," he said. "Researchers have found chemical and physical evidence supporting something we've known all along: Your mind and body are closely linked. *What happens in the mind is inevitably re-*

170

flected in the health or disease of the body."

The moment I walked in the door, Mary took a look at me and said, "I can see you won't be very good dinner company tonight."

"Uh, what's that?" I asked. "What did you say?"

She laughed. "Bob, I can tell when something big's going on in your mind . . . I can tell that your thoughts are a million miles away from the table . . ."

"Is it that obvious?"

"Of course. And it's alright." She hugged me and shooed me out of the kitchen. "Go wash up. I'll deliver your dinner to you on a tray. Then you can stay right with whatever it is until you get it all sorted out. I love you."

"Thanks, Hon. I do need some time alone . . ."

I ate mechanically, my mind wrestling with Dr. Fox's thesis. He spoke of anger, rage, frustration, bitterness, fear embarrassment and other negative emotions and the effect they have upon our bodies.

If we cling to these negative feelings, Fox said, cuddle them, fondle them, culture them, and make them a part of our personality, they will actually prompt "the manufacture and release of (what he called) chemical messengers that travel to every part of (one's) body, spreading the bad news."

Thoughts in one's mind become adrenaline, noradrenaline, cortisone, ACTH, and other chemical substances in the body *that alter the delicate biochemical balance of the body and weaken the immune system.*

And when this happens to a person he becomes prey to all kinds of diseases that he would ordinarily shrug off.

"Wow!" I said, nearly dumping my empty dishes upon the floor. "AIDS doesn't kill people. I've been saying that for weeks."

It was becoming clearer and clearer to me:

AIDS is the effect, *not the cause.*

AIDS reflects and displays the destroyed immune system, but *AIDS does not cause the immune breakdown.*

When the immune system has been made inoperative by renegade chemicals released by uncontrolled negativity, the result is a body that is left defenseless and unable to protect itself. The result: it becomes host to all manner of so-called "opportunistic" diseases, such as Kaposi's sarcoma, pneumocystis carinii and certain cancers.

Death, when it comes, is blamed upon AIDS, which is unfair. AIDS did not cause the death. AIDS cannot cause anything. AIDS is merely the condition the body finds itself in when it (the body) has destroyed its own immune system!

There, I had it!

I remembered the day I had reacted so violently to the radio preacher who had declared that AIDS was God's judgment upon our wicked world.

Tonight, more clearly than ever before, I realized how wrong, how simplistic, how *wickedly controlling* that theological or philosophical position was. AIDS, in my opinion, was no more than the result of breaking God's immutable laws. Even as one would be "punished" by recklessly violating the laws of gravity or electricity, so would one be punished by violating the laws that had to do with the caring of one's body.

"Stress is the reaction of your body, mind, or spirit to the facts (that impinge upon our lives)," Dr. Fox said. "You choose the reaction; it's not forced upon you by the hand of God."

It's our reactions, our attitudes, our *thoughts*, I realized, that are the "stressostats" of our bodies. Thoughts produce things. And "the things they produce," said Dr. Fox, "are the chemical substances such as adrenaline and ACTH. When one's thoughts produce these things at the wrong time, in such excessive amounts, *the result is a battered immune system*.

"Your thoughts have produced such things in you. That's why you are sick."

Bitterness, then, I thought, *anger and hostility, relentless pressure of competition, aggressiveness, unreleased or unforgiven memories of abuse and/or molestation as children, fear, in short, all unrelieved tensions, frustrations and emotions, automatically produce an overabundance of chemicals in our bodies that bring about the breakdown or total destruction of our immune systems.*

The picture was coming clear to me:

External drugs are chemicals. Wrongly used (or abused) they bring harm to the body.

By the same token, *internal drugs (which our bodies produce) are also chemicals*. They, too, when wrongly produced and used (or abused), bring harm to the body.

This was making more and more sense.

Seeking the primal root cause of AIDS and *all* disease, I began boiling down all my known facts and information to the lowest common denominator. As I did, I arrived at what I believe is a fundamental premise: Both hard drugs (externally ingested or injected) and "soft" drugs (internally produced and "injected"), bring progressive destruction to various organs of the body, which is the real cause of all sickness.

Which we call disease.

If this is true, then all diseases—whether we "name" them the flu, asthma, cancer, arthritis, osteoporosis, diabetes, or AIDS—are but artificial labels randomly-placed upon various sets of "symptoms" depending upon their physical location. And all diseases are nothing but drug-induced, progressive toxemia (or poison), either endogenous (internally generated) or exogenous (externally generated).

And when the unrelieved toxemia gets bad enough, the immune system begins to self-destruct. AIDS, I realized, coming full circle in my reasoning, does not destroy the immune system. AIDS is the result, the final result of a destroyed immune system.

Which is the reason why AIDS is always fatal: the body has reached the end of its resources to reconstruct or rejuvenate itself. It has no place else to go.

Except to die.

What about Roger?

Why did his immune system begin functioning again?

This answer seemed clear to me now.

By fasting, Roger's body was able to eliminate the stored-up drugs he had accumulated. By placing him in a stress-free environment with caring people, the self-induced drugs that his fears and anger had produced for years were also eliminated.

Ellen, too, had replaced Roger's loneliness with acceptance and happiness. Given such an environment, Roger's body had been able to do the rest, and heal itself.

However, I thought, *there is doubtless a point of no return in any body, beyond which it can no longer reverse the inevitable destructive results of a failed immune system. And that must come when a body's degeneration has reached a point where tissue has been broken down and actually destroyed. At that juncture it would be beyond even the body's remarkable regenerative powers to heal itself . . .*

But how, I wondered, could any doctor, a mere human who is certainly not God, make the determination for another, as to when or at what point his body has reached such a condition? Despite that doctor's skill and training, the answer was, to me, crystal clear: It is not possible!

It was late when I reached these conclusions, but I had to share them with somebody. I tapped on Roger's door.

"Come in," he said immediately.

Roger was sitting up in bed. Ellen was sitting next to him. The glow on their faces revealed the mutuality of their feelings for each other. I felt like an intruder. "Excuse me," I said, and turned to go.

"No, Bob," Roger said. "Please come in. We have an important announcement to make . . ."

I sat on the end of his bed. "Let me guess."

Ellen blushed. Roger asked, "Is it that obvious?"

I nodded. "Yes. And I sincerely congratulate both of you."

"I believe my physical crisis is past," Roger said. "And I really think that I'm well on my way to complete recovery. Don't you agree?"

"Yes, Roger. I am in full agreement. And I am so very happy for you. For you, Roger . . . and for you, Ellen."

Ellen spoke then. "Doctor Smith, we want to thank you for the part you played in bringing healing to Roger . . . and for bringing us together."

I acknowledged her thanks with a nod and a smile.

"Now, Bob," Roger said, "I believe you, too, have an important announcement."

"Yes, but it might be a little involved to get into this late at night."

"Does it concern AIDS . . . and me?"

"Yes. I've finally got it all clear in my head."

"What's that?"

"My thinking concerning the how and why you have regained your health . . ."

Roger settled back. Ellen sat close to him, gently stroking his hand. Roger said, "Then tell us, Bob . . . because now," he smiled at Ellen, "our prospects are bright, and we've got all the time in the world . . ."

CHAPTER TWENTY ONE

Despite my success with Roger Cochran, and my determination of what I now believed to be the actual etiology of AIDS, two powerful concerns, yes fears, were beginning to form within me, neither of which I could either adequately validate, or shake.

First, based upon my assumption that AIDS was the *result* and not the cause of AIDS, it was inconceivable to me that some, if not many others who had access to the same information had not arrived at the same conclusion. And if that were the case, I wondered if I was the first or only scientist to have actually demonstrated in a living human "laboratory" that it is possible to rejuvenate a human immune system, and thus return a condemned AIDS patient to a condition of life and vibrant health.

Were there others who had wrestled with the same problems and arrived at the same conclusions as I? And if so, had they begun applying those same life-giving principles to the treatment of other diseases? Or had they, because of medical establishment peer pressure, fear, or economic reasons, ignored their findings and continued to practice in their usual orthodox manner?

Were there yet others who had glimpsed the truth as I had seen it and who had chosen to capitalize on the ignorance of the masses by building financially-powerful pharmaceutical or health-care empires?

As I mulled over this possibility I chanced across a letter to the editor of INSIGHT magazine (August 1986), written by Dr. Stephen S. Caiazza, who was Chairman of the New York Committee of Concerned Physicians. In his letter, Dr. Caiazza said, "AIDS is becoming big business, involving *billions of dollars* in potential profits for the biomedical industry. . . ."

This fact alone disturbed me greatly. But there was more.

"However," Dr. Caiazzo went on, "because of the fierce competition within the industry, it is no longer unusual for those of us intimately involved with AIDS to be offered insider information, stock advice, 'consultant' fees, etc., in appreciation for being supportive of a company's new and potentially lucrative therapeutic or diagnostic modality. No doctor worthy of his degree could possibly accept such an offer. It would be a violation of all standard medical ethics."

I was in total agreement with Dr. Caiazzo's stance.

"The issue, though," he went on, "runs still deeper. Due to the limited and extremely difficult manner in which it is transmitted, AIDS is fundamentally a disease of behavior. With proper health policies at all levels, sound education of all Americans and appropriate individual responsibility, *AIDS is essentially 100% preventable.*"

"Dear God!" I said to Mary, who peeked into my office at that moment, "here's an eminent and powerful physician who believes AIDS can be prevented!"

In my excitement to make such a discover, I was nervously pacing the room, waving my magazine in the air.

"That *is* wonderful!" Mary agreed, and gave me a hug before going down the hall. When I could settle down to do so, I read the rest of the letter.

"By analogy," the doctor continued, "it belongs in the same category as smoking-induced lung cancer, or death and injury resulting from drunk driving.

"Thus, when companies like Genetech ignore prevention and talk instead about developing a vaccine against an avoidable disease and recruit prestigious doctors and researchers as 'consultants' to facilitate their image while, simultaneously, *their stock is selling at 265 times earnings*, one must be skeptical. Are we hearing expert science and medicine, or are we hearing expert public relations?"

I groaned in frustration. To think that professional people were actually capable of capitalizing on human misery to such an extent. It was at such times that I was embarrassed to be called a physician.

Dr. Caiazzo concluded his letter with a powerful paragraph:

"AIDS is a human tragedy of unbelievable proportions," he wrote. "*It is also a disease we can put an end to as soon as we find the will and determination to do so. I fear, though, that such a commitment will never be realized, given the industry that we see spawning around AIDS.*"

As I read Dr. Caiazzo's concluding sentence, I felt the same cold righteous anger I had felt in Viet Nam when I was being called upon to mend the blasted, burned and torn bodies of my own countrymen who were being slaughtered in a useless, hopeless conflict that had not even been dignified to be called a war.

"*We are very close to the irrevocable time,*" Dr. Caiazzo said, "*when we will need AIDS and be unable to do without it because it will be essential to the earnings of too many companies.*"

"Dear God," I said to nobody in particular, "can it be true that we have prostituted ourselves to the point that the immeasurable suffering of our fellow men means nothing to us except a few more dollars?"

Throughout my medical career, I had been loyal to the AMA and my fellow physicians. But lately, because of all my research—much of it having to do with what the AMA calls "alternative" approaches—I was beginning to think there must be many other ways and means of treating patients beside the "acceptable" orthodox means of drugs, surgery and radiation.

There were times when I was finding myself adrift on a sea of unanswered questions.

And it was at just such times, that when I read items like Dr. Caiazza's letter, I began finding myself questioning not just the validity of the "AIDS industry," but of the entire medical profession.

Even before reading Dr. Caiazzo's letter I'd been asking myself, "Why are we being bombarded with AIDS PR material at every turn?" I was often staggered at the sheer immensity of the AIDS blitzkreig. It was impossible to avoid the constant media barrage.

"It's too much, too soon," I told David Cohen. "It's as though we're being deluged with AIDS hype in such quantities for a purpose . . ."

"I agree," David said. "But for what purpose?"

"To prevent us from thinking rationally about it."

He just stared at me. "But, why?"

I shook my head. "I don't know. I just don't know.

But I intend to find out."

I had already come to the conclusion that the so-called "AIDS symptoms" were not new. There had always been symptoms that were now being defined as AIDS symptoms. Personally I even wondered about the "statistical increase" of such symptoms. Could this be attributed to better reporting?

Or could it be, and the very thought chilled me to the bone, that diseases that had once been called something else were now being lumped together and called AIDS? If that were the case, then it would most surely indicate a massive manipulation of the whole medical institution.

Gradually there was growing within me the awful feeling that the "AIDS industry" was nothing more than just that: an industry. One that had been created for the single, or at least the primary purpose, of making money—lots of money—for the drug and medical establishment.

And if that was the case, which I was beginning to believe, then *it meant that AIDS, per se, was a cruel hoax.*

Is that possible? No, I thought, that's too monstrous. Too unthinkable!

But, perhaps it is not so unthinkable. Hasn't history shown us that it is possible for a tiny handful of politically and money minded persons possessed of enormous financial resources to perpetrate monstrous lies of such dimensions so as to have been believed and accepted?

Even though the thought was "unthinkable," I sat there thinking it just the same.

It was very plain to me that the medical profession, including myself, had not actually had anything to do with Roger's return to health. Roger's body, when

provided with the opportunity, had done the job itself! Doctors and drugs had not been needed. X-rays
and hospitals, with their huge facilities and staffs had
not been utilized.

Yet prior to Roger's dramatic return to health he
had been drained by the medical profession.

They had accepted his money, sliced him open with
scalpels, poked him full of holes into which they had
poured drugs and from which they had drained
blood. They had practiced their deadly game of drugging upon him until it became clear that nothing
worked.

They had failed. Yet they were unwilling to accept
biological alternatives as viable options.

Instead, they had made their full and final decision:
They declared him "untouchable," tacked a "terminal"
label upon him and shoved him out into the cold.

From that point, Roger's only future was the grave.

As a medical man myself, I knew that all physicians were not so crass. I knew that there were thousands of compassionate and concerned doctors who
were pouring out their energies to keep their patients
alive and well.

But it now seemed obvious to me that AIDS, per
se, was much more than just another disease, or epidemic. It was an institution. A carefully designed institution. And that behind the "AIDS scare" there
was a huge and powerful money machine that was
calling the shots and controlling the entire pharmaceutical and health-care industry. An article in the
Los Angeles Herald Examiner (March 21, 1987)
served to add fuel to my thinking. Speaking of the
drug, Retrovir, made by Burroughs Wellcome Company, the manufacturer estimated "that annual treat-

ment costs would be $8,000 to $10,000 a patient. . . ."

Eight to ten thousand dollars per year, per AIDS patient!

These and other facts led me to believe that men like myself and thousands of other well-meaning medical professionals were being unconscionably manipulated to do their bidding. And for the most part we had fallen for their propaganda and had played their game.

This was indeed monstrous.

Oh, God, I agonized, *if there is a hell, those who have reaped their pound of flesh from the agonized cries of the living dead should be mummified in their money and forced to suffer forever!*

CHAPTER
TWENTY TWO

I was standing face-to-face with a very serious consideration: Based on what I now believe, can I retain my integrity and stand by my principles and not succumb to the pressure of orthodox medicine? Could that pressure become so great that I would crumble? Or, worse yet, if I attempted to stand by my own principles, would I simply be destroyed by the sheer power of orthodoxy?

I knew I did not have the resources to stand against the combined forces of orthodox medicine. Yet, I wasn't willing to give up my hold on biological medicine, which I now believed would become the medical wave of the future. What could I do?

I was hoping that I could convince both David and Roger to help me develop the therapy that had worked so well on Roger. I longed to research the finer points of biological medicine and to begin using it on other patients. Not just AIDS patients, but most patients.

"Frankly, though," I was telling Mary, "it really scares me to think about launching out."

"Why, Bob? You're young enough. You have a solid practice. You're well accepted in a number of hospitals . . ."

"There's more to it than that," I told her. "Lately I've been reading of several physicians who moved out, to use your term, into 'alternative' approaches to healing. And several of them ran into difficulties . . ."

"Difficulties? In what way?" she asked, genuinely puzzled.

"Well, when doctors disagree with AMA standards of medicine and thus violate their accepted procedures, the AMA, the Federal Drug Administration, the National Cancer Institute, and other agencies go after them . . ."

"Go after them? What does that mean?"

"For one, they harrass the man until he comes into line. If he doesn't get the message, they take him to court and close him down. Or even worse."

"That's really hard to believe," Mary said. "You mean to say the American Medical Association would do that?"

"You bet your boots. And the Federal agencies as well. Let me give you a for instance. There's Dr. Lawrence Burton, who had a clinic in Freeport, in the Bahamas."

"What happened to him?"

"To begin with U.S. medical authorities drove Dr. Burton out of Long Island, New York. Then when he opened up a clinic in the Bahamas and continued to treat patients with his immuno-augmentive therapy, U.S. authorities closed down his clinic."

"But, why?"

"Simply because Burton was using alternative means of treating patients. And the AMA wouldn't allow it."

"But I don't understand, Bob . . ."

"Neither do I, Hon. But it happens all the time. As recently as March of last year, a Dr. Bruce Halstead, right here in Southern California, was sentenced to four years in state prison and had his medical license revoked."

Mary gasped. "But what for?"

"The only charges against him had to do with practicing alternative medicine, something the AMA won't countenance."

"I had no idea . . ."

"See that pile of clippings on my credenza? It represents scores of doctors, osteopaths, chiropractors, nutritionists, and other health-oriented professionals who are being sued by the AMA, the Federal Drug Administration, the National Cancer Institute and other government agencies on trumped up charges. Though there have been abuses in the field, and these agencies are on the lookout for quackery, *many of these people being sued are qualified, ethical, thinking men and women* who have their patients' health in mind."

I sighed. "So you can see why it really scares me to think of launching out and using some new or different approaches."

Nevertheless, I was determined to keep the ball rolling as far as my new understanding was concerned. I knew I couldn't do it alone, so I decided to discuss it with David.

"By now it's clear that Roger is doing great, that he's on the way to total wellness . . ." I began at our next meeting.

David took another bite of his salad and nodded. "Yes, his recovery is amazing. He's the only AIDS patient I've heard of who has made it."

"There certainly must be others," I said, "but I agree. I don't personally know of any. And all the statistics prophesy certain death for anyone with AIDS."

David finished his lunch and leaned back. "I take it you've got something important to discuss?"

"Right. In a word, where do we go from here?"

"I've been wondering about that. I'm with you. For a while—quite a while, in fact—I was skeptical. I never hid that from you. You knew how I felt all along."

"Right. And I appreciate that." I finished my last bite of salad and nodded for the waiter to bring the tab. "I've got some ideas that I'd like to bounce off you . . ."

He checked his watch. "Go ahead. We've still got over half an hour."

"Well, to begin with, David, I'm quite excited about Roger's evident return to good health . . ." He nodded, but I went on. "And I'd like very much to continue working in the AIDS area. To test some of my new thinking . . . to do some writing . . ."

David frowned slightly. "At this point are you thinking of 'going public' with all this?"

"No. Not at all. In fact, I don't want to even hint at any advertising campaign. If AIDS patients come, we'll treat them. If not, I'll use the same approach on other complaints."

David relaxed visibly. "That's good, Bob. Because, to do with other patients what you did with Roger would be, to say the least, difficult. If not impossible." He frowned. "Another thing, Bob, we don't even know for certain if the biological approach will work with everybody."

"I agree. I think it will depend upon the deterioration of both the immune system as well as the patient himself. If there has been serious tissue damage, I have some doubts about the ability of the body to bring about total wellness as Roger's body was able to do."

I handed the waiter my credit card.

"And something else I know you've thought about. We certainly don't have the facilities. But, I believe there are some such facilities around . . ."

"You do?" He raised his eyebrows. "I've never heard of any."

"There are health centers that specialize in fasting and nutrition. Facilities run by doctors or nutrition-ists . . ."

"Not run by quacks?"

"Right. I already know of a couple. But there are many others, and of course I'd check them out thor-oughly before I assigned a patient to them. But, the problem is, I can't run a practice and run around checking them out?"

"Nor can I," David said slowly. "Any ideas?"

"Yes, I do. I was thinking of Roger."

"Roger? Hmmm. Hadn't thought of that. What would you have him do? Have you talked to him yet?"

"Second question first. No, I haven't even hinted anything to him. I wanted to discuss it with you first. I thought we could have him go around, check out facilities, personnel, and so on. Then, very carefully, cautiously, begin sending patients—AIDS patients, arthritic patients, maybe even heart patients—to one or more of those health centers. And Roger would supervise that part of our wellness program. What do you think?"

David smiled for the first time. "Excellent idea. As

189

a former AIDS patient, he'd be able to handle it. I'm for it."

"I'm glad you like the idea, David. Now, why don't I discuss the matter with him, get his thinking, then all of us get together and brainstorm . . .?"

The timing seemed right. By now Roger was gaining weight rapidly, along with a vibrancy of body and spirit I had known in him years ago. When I told Mary of the conference with David, she said, "Let's go for a weekend on the boat . . ."

It was sunup on a Saturday morning. And the four of us, Mary and I, Ellen and Roger had just cleared the Marina Del Rey breakwater, headed for Catalina. Resplendent in her new coat of paint, the little schooner, "BandAid," which David and I owned co-operatively, seemed glad to strut her stuff. The wind was abaft the beam; the swells were light. We hoisted both the mains'l and the jib, then relaxed to enjoy the trip.

Mary and Ellen were in the galley preparing a late breakfast. Roger and I were in the cockpit, with him at the wheel. It was a perfect setting to discuss the future.

Preamble to what I had in mind, I asked, "Roger, have you thought what you might be doing?"

"Doing when?" he asked with a twinkle.

"Well . . . well, when you get settled. And after . . ."

"After the wedding?" he chuckled. He and Ellen had announced their wedding for mid summer.

"Yes, of course. I wouldn't expect a courting man to do anything so menial as work."

After a few minutes of banter, Roger studied the set of the main sail seriously before speaking. "Actually, Bob, Ellen and I have done a great deal of thinking about, as you put it, the future."

The wind changed and Roger eased up the wheel to fill the sail. "And, Bob, to put it succinctly, and bluntly, I don't have a lot of ready cash." He grinned lopsidedly. "Or any other kind of cash . . ."

We both laughed. "As you might expect, I'd spent about every dime I had by the time I dragged into your office that day."

"Yeah, I surmised as much."

"And," he said, looking me straight in the eye, "frankly, I'm in the market for a job . . . are you interested?"

"In you? Or in a job?"

"Touche! In a job for me . . ." Roger had been at the wheel since we undocked and I could see he was getting tired.

"Like me to take it for a while?" I asked.

He nodded and relinquished the wheel then comfortably seated himself in the lee cockpit. "I'm serious, Bob. I'm serious in wanting to go back to work. I'm about ready now. And . . ." he paused meditatively, "Ellen and I have talked this over. After all, it should be a joint decision . . . and, it's our combined opinion that I should be working with you and David. And . . ."

Roger paused in mid sentence.

"And . . . what?" I asked.

"And I'd like to continue the work on AIDS that you—that is, we, but mostly you—have just begun." He looked at me expectantly. "What do you say? How about it?"

I held the wheel with two fingers and reached across. "Put her there, Roger . . . welcome aboard as my new partner."

"What do you mean?"

"David and I have just been waiting for you to speak up, to say something . . ."

Roger began to speak, but I held my hand up. "Wait just a minute. I want to tell you what we had in mind. Then you can consider it. Fair enough?"

"Fair," Roger said, but I could tell he was eager to accept.

"What I—and, well, David, too, but at this point it's more my idea than his—right in line with what you just said, want to continue utilizing what I'm calling our 'wellness treatment' philosophy. Biological medicine." I frowned. "The AMA calls it 'alternative medicine.' Anyway we want to work with any AIDS victims, that is *if* they come . . ."

"It's inevitable," Roger broke in.

"But we'll also be using the same methods of treatment on other patients. Arthritic patients . . . I told you how well Glenda is feeling, didn't I?"

"Yes. And she looks good."

"Heart patients, diabetics. Patients with all kinds of complaints. We'll do this very slowly at first, and try not to attract the attention of some of the AMA diehards. Know what I mean?"

"I know. Some medical heretics—and that's what you'd be called—are hounded out of their practices. Some even jailed. Yes, Bob, I know what you're talking about."

"It could be risky, Roger. I want you to know that. Some doctors are losing their licenses . . ."

He nodded slowly. "I know that, Bob. I know. But I figure I've been resurrected . . . and orthodox medicine didn't do it. I was nearly dead from orthodoxy when I came to you. It was you, Bob, who dared to do something different. If it hadn't been for you and

192

your courage, I'd . . . well, I'd be dead by now . . ."

Roger glanced down the hatch and watched Ellen and Mary preparing our meal. When he turned back, his jaw was set. "Bob, I didn't really have much to live for before. Now I do. You stuck your neck out for me. And I . . . well, anyway . . ."

He cleared his throat and wiped his cheeks with his hand. "I just want to say . . . count me in. All the way. Okay?"

"That's what I thought you'd say, Roger. And I'm really pleased with your decision. But, let me finish telling you what I had in mind . . . I know of some health centers . . . some of which I think we could use for patient referral. Under our supervision, of course. Maybe later we'd even purchase the centers . . ."

The wind was freshening. "Give me a hand with the main," I said, "let's reef it a little."

Ten minutes later we were bowling along at a sharp clip. "I mentioned all of this to David. And we've agreed, that if this suits your fancy, we'd like for you to spearhead that effort. Are you interested? Or, do you want to think about it?"

Roger stood so suddenly that he almost struck his head on the boom. "Interested? *Interested*? That's almost exactly what I told Ellen I'd like to be doing. Sign me on!"

The timing was perfect. Mary appeared in the hatch and clanged the ship's bell eight times. "Eight bells, and all is well, Captain," she said, with a smiling salute. "And, incidentally, breakfast is ready."

CHAPTER
TWENTY THREE

David and I were in my office when Roger's call
came. "I'm at the center," he said, "and it's beautiful!"
"Which one?" I asked.
"The one run by Hastings. You know, the chiro-
practor."
"Oh, yes, that's where Glenda went. Tell me about
it."
I motioned for David to get on the other line. As
he picked up the receiver, Roger was saying, ". . . the
grounds are heavily wooded . . . individual cabins for
one or two. Each with its own kitchen and private
bath. Fireplace. Central dining hall. The place is well
cared for."
"How many will the center accommodate?" David
asked.
"Dr. Hastings told me the private cabins will house
fifty. And the lodge will handle another forty. Oh,
yes, there's a private cabin for the director . . . another for the maintenance crew . . ."
"What about Hastings' assistants?" I asked.

Roger's voice was clear and crisp. "There are four of them," he said. "They all house in a duplex, two to each apartment."

"One more question," I said, "what's happening at the center? How is Hastings doing?"

"That's the problem," Roger said.

"What do you mean?" David asked.

"Well, the AMA is trying to close him down. They've got a lawsuit pending against him?"

"A lawsuit?" I said. "What are the charges?"

"Practicing medicine without a license."

David and I looked at each other. David spoke first. "Can they substantiate the charges?"

"Not as far as I can see," Roger said. "Hastings doesn't even practice chiropractics here. He's got an RN to register the clients—he doesn't use the term patient. He doesn't treat anybody . . . for anything . . ."

"Then how? . . . I don't understand . . ." I said.

"Neither does he, Bob. He's very frustrated. The charges are ambiguous . . . but it looks like they're out to get him?"

"But, why?" David broke in. "Why?"

Roger sighed to vent his own frustration. "The only reason I can think of . . . and Hastings, too . . . is that *sick people*, I mean *really* sick people are coming here. And when they leave here they are well . . ."

"What kind of sick people?" I asked. Along with sharing the frustration Roger felt, for himself as well as Hastings, I was beginning to feel excitement well up within me.

"Well, when I told Hastings about my own situation . . . about having AIDS, and how I'm now completely well and healthy, he, well, he just nodded. He told me, 'I know. Happens all the time. We had three people with AIDS here last month. When they went home I suggested they make an appointment with a different doctor. To go in for an examination *without telling him anything* about the previous diagnosis . . .' "

"And did they do that?" David asked.

"They sure did!"

"And . . .?" I asked.

"Hastings told me that every one of those clients took his advice and did as he suggested. Now, here's the wonderful part: In each case the doctor gave them a clean bill of health!"

Roger paused to catch his breath. I heard David breathe, "Wow!"

"And that's not all, men." Roger went on. "Hastings opened his records to me. I saw them, read them. They read like a report on Our Lady of Lourdes. All kinds of people have been to the center. Some who couldn't walk, arthritics. Even worse. Not everybody is well when they leave. But many of them are . . . lots of them. Even so," Roger added thoughtfully, "the percentage of those who leave Hastings' center in good health is higher than those who leave most hospitals in good health . . .

"But, perhaps even more important, the percentage of those who *stay* in good health remains higher . . ."

"Why is that, Roger?" David asked.

"Because, while they are at the center they are educated, not just on the subject of how to get well and stay well, but concerning what caused them to become ill in the first place."

"So they receive lasting benefit from the experience," I said, thinking, *What a wonderful gift to those people.*

"Yes, the benefits are literally both life and health

changing," Roger agreed.

"When they leave the center in a well condition, who verifies their healing?" David asked.

"Not Hastings. Nor the RN. They tell the clients to go back to their own doctors for examination. And that's what they do."

Nobody spoke for a moment. All we could hear was the sound of our breathing. Finally I asked, "What do you think, Roger?"

"You mean about setting up a center like this. Or trying to buy one and run it?"

"Either one."

Roger replied carefully, as though he'd given plenty of thought to his answer. "I don't think it'll work. I think the AMA would soon be after us, too?"

"On what charges?" David asked. "We're doctors, MD's."

"I know," Roger said. "Hastings and I talked about that for a long time. He said the AMA is cracking down on any operation that even looks like it's using an alternative approach. He told me they're closing clinics and private operations all over the country. He's frustrated. And scared . . ."

After Roger hung up David and I just sat and looked at each other for a long moment. David just shook his head.

"It isn't fair, David," I said, "not fair at all . . . people are dying from lack of knowledge. And they don't know how to help themselves . . ."

"I know, Bob. I know. How well I know. We've gone over this territory before . . . for hours at a time." David absentmindedly shined the toe of one shoe on his pant leg. When he looked up he asked pointedly, "What are you going to do, Bob?"

"There's only one thing left to do," I told him. "Write a book . . . tell the people that *there is* good news. Good news about AIDS. Good news about most of their ailments. And that there is a way . . .."

"But what good will that do?" David asked.

"Find a publisher with the guts to publish such a book. Get it into the hands of the people . . ." I was pacing the floor.

"Because, the way I see it, the only way for us to see a change is for it to come from the people. Let them start a mighty ground swell of . . . of anger . . . frustration. Get them to demand changes in the medical profession. In the hospitals and health-care industry . . ."

David was on his feet now. "That's right, Bob. If the people make enough noise they'll get the attention of the lawmakers. And if the lawmakers have got to get things changed in order to get elected, things *will* change!"

Janine tapped at the door and peeked in. "Dr. Bob, you have a patient in the examining room . . . an AIDS patient . . ."

David and I looked at each other. I arose and followed Janine.

The man was smaller than Roger, and younger, but he wore the same hangdog look of desperation on his face. And something else. Guilt? Shame? Resignation. It was all there, and more. The look I'd seen so often in the eyes of patients who had been told they were terminally ill.

"I've got AIDS," he said, and his lips quivered. "I'm going to die . . ."

I wheeled my chair over to him. His face wore a gray pallor.

199

"Why do you think you're going to die?"

He shrugged. "They all do."

"They do?" My question seemed to startle him.

"Don't they?" he asked quickly. "That's what everybody says."

I looked at his folder. "No, Mr. Allen, they don't all die."

For a brief instant I caught a flicker of hope in his eyes. "Are you sure?"

"Yes, Mr. Allen, I'm sure . . ."

He stared at me uncomprehendingly.

"Do you really want to get well?"

"Yes . . . yes. Yes! But there's no vaccine . . . and some say there won't be for years . . ." His words became a sob. "Oh, yes, Doctor, I want to live. *I want to live!*"

"Mr. Allen, your body wants to live, too. But your body is sick. You know that. And to make you well again, we've got to work on both your body *and* your mind."

His eyes were fixed on mine. "I . . . I . . . I'm not sure I understand. Please tell me again . . ."

"Mr. Allen, you are sick because some things you have done and the way you have lived have damaged your immune system. You have hurt it so badly that it's almost given up. Understand?"

He nodded slowly. "I . . . I think so."

"So, Mr. Allen, if we—you and I—can assist your immune system to begin functioning again, then you'll get well . . ."

"But there's no drug yet, no vaccine that can do that . . ."

I gripped the man by both his shoulders. "Listen to me. All a drug can do is make you more comfortable.

Temporarily. For a little while. But the drug can't heal you. Only your body can do that . . ."

The man was hanging upon every word.

". . . And if I can help you to stop doing the things that hurt your immune system . . . then there's a chance that you can get well."

The patient's slumped shoulders straightened. "What can I do, Doctor? I'll do anything. *Anything*!"

"I will tell you what to do. But first I want you to know that it's going to be a tough, uphill fight. Very tough. But if you will hang in there . . . and do *exactly* what I tell you to do, then, together . . . we just might be able to lick this thing. And get you well."

Tears began coursing down his cheeks. "I've been going from doctor to doctor . . . and hospital to hospital for months. For months, Doctor! And why . . . why, oh, why hasn't anyone else told me this . . .?"

A WORD FROM ROGER . . .

Although almost all of the material in this book has come from the files, publications and personal interviews of informed health services practitioners and scientists, we want to remind you that you should not consider the material in this book to be the practice of medicine.

However, the information in this book has been provided with the understanding that you may act on it at your own risk, taking full responsibility for your own personal health and well being; a concept which coincides with the personal responsibility you accept when you enter any health-care facility and before you undergo any surgical procedure.

Because of the persecution experienced by professionals who utilize non-toxic alternative healthcare methods and procedures, many of these individuals, including Dr. Bob and myself, have tended to project a low profile, for their own economic, emotional and physical safety. This fact makes it difficult for me to answer those of you who keep asking, "How do I find knowledgeable, credible healthcare facilities in my area?"

In order for you to receive that information openly, in keeping with your constitutional right to freely choose your own healthcare, we strongly recommend that, individually, or in concert with advocates of alternative healthcare, you petition your political representatives to enact or amend laws which will make alternative options available.

If you feel you require opinions, diagnoses, treatments, therapeutic advice, correction of your lifestyle, or any other assistance relating to your health, and wish to investigate some alternative treatment institutions and/or health-care professionals, it is your constitutional right to do so. To assist you in this endeavor, I suggest you contact Project CURE and the National Health Federation. Both organizations are actively engaged in keeping their constituents informed regarding orthodox medicine's self-serving attempts to pass laws limiting individuals from freely choosing their own health-care services. Both are also involved in enlisting the support of all interested U.S. citizens in preventing the passage of such laws. Their addresses are:

Project CURE, 2020 K Street, N.W., Suite 350
Washington, D.C. 20069

National Health Federation, 212 W. Foothill Blvd.,
Monrovia, CA 91016

These two organizations are but two of the many groups that are working toward this cause, but they will give you a place to begin asking your questions. Furthermore, they will both help keep you informed concerning these vital issues as well as instruct you in getting actively involved in letter-writing campaigns that will make a difference.

On a personal level, thanks to a doctor who was willing to put his practice and his future on the line for me, I am a well man today. Now we are working hard together to open the doors to alternative health care, so that other informed doctors won't run the risk of laying their futures on the line to freely treat their patients, and to make it possible for you to make your own personal healthcare choice.

We can't do all this alone. We need your help. This you can do by contacting one or both of the agencies above and requesting information. Then, fully informed, begin contacting and airing your opinions with your state and federal representatives.

—Roger Cochran, M.D.

SUGGESTED READING

Airola, Paavo O., N.D., *There IS a Cure for Arthritis*. West Nyack, New York: Parker Publishing Co., Inc., 1968.

Airola, Paavo O., Ph.D., N.D., *Cancer, Causes, Prevention and Treatment, The Total Approach*. Phoenix, Arizona: Health Plus, Publishers. 1963.

Allen, Hannah, *Don't Get Stuck, The Case Against Vaccinations and Injections*. Oldsmar, Florida: Natural Hygiene Press, 1985.

Antonio, Gene, *The AIDS Cover-Up?*. San Francisco: Ignatius Press, 1986.

Barnhart, Edward R., Publisher, *Physicians' Desk Reference, 41 Edition*. Oradell, N.J.: Medical Economics Company, Inc., 1987.

Benson, Herbert, M.D., with William Proctor, *Beyond the Relaxation Response*. New York: Berkley Books, 1986.

Benson, Herbert, M.D., with Miriam Z. Klipper, *The Relaxation Response*. New York: Avon Books, 1976.

Berkow, Robert, M.D., Editor-in-Chief, *The Merck Manual of Diagnosis and Therapy, Fourteenth Edi-*

tion. Rahway, N.J.: Merck Sharp & Dohme Research Laboratories, 1982.

Black, David, *The Plague Years, A Chronicle of AIDS, The Epidemic of Our Times.* New York: Simon and Schuster, 1985.

Bliznakov, Emile G., M.D. and Gerald L. Hunt, *The Miracle Nutrient Coenzyme Q10.* New York: Bantam Books, 1987.

Bragg, Paul C., N.D., Ph.D., and Patricia Bragg, N.D., Ph.D., *The Miracle of Fasting.* Santa Barbara, California: Health Science, 1985.

Buttram, Harold E., M.D., *Vaccinations and Immune Malfunction.* Quakertown, PA: The Humanitarian Publishing Company, 1985.

✳ Cantwell, Alan, Jr., M.D., *AIDS, The Mystery and The Solution.* Los Angeles: Aires Rising Press, 1986.

Cawood, Gayle, M.Ed., Janice McCall Failes and Frank W. Cawood, *Prescription Drug Encyclopedia.* Peachtree City, GA: F C & A, Inc., 1986

Chase, Allan, King K. Holmes, Per-Anders Mardh, and Paul J. Wiesner, *The Truth About STD.* New York: William Morrow & Company, Inc., 1983.

Diamond, Harvey and Marilyn, *Fit for Life.* New York: Warner Books, 1985.

Elben, *Vaccination Condemned.* Los Angeles: Better Life Research, 1981.

Fry, T.C. "The Great AIDS Hysteria," *Healthful Living,* October, November, December, 1985, Life Science Institute, 6600 Burleson Road, Austin, TX 78744.

Giller, Robert M., M.D. and Kathy Matthews, *Medical Makeover.* New York: Warner Books, 1986.

Govoni, Laura E., Ph.D., R.N., and Janice E. Hayes, Ph.D., R.N., *Drugs and Nursing Implications, Edition 4.* Norwalk, Connecticut: Appleton-

Century-Crofts, 1982.

Illich, Ivan, *Medical Nemesis, The Expropriation of Health*. New York: Pantheon Books, 1976.

McCall, Fr. Peter, OMF Cap., and Maryanne Lacy, *An Invitation To Healing*. Yonkers, New York: The House of Peace, 1985.

McDougall, John A., M.D., and Mary A. McDougall, *The MacDougall Plan*. Piscataway, N.J.: New Century Publishers, Inc., 1983.

Mendelsohn, Robert S., M.D., *Confessions of a Medical Heretic*. New York: Warner Books, 1979.

Nolen, William A., *The Making of a Surgeon*. New York: Random House, Inc., 1968.

Oswald, Jean A., and Herbert M. Shelton, Ph.D., *Fasting for the Health of It*. Pueblo, Colorado: Nationwide Press, Ltd., 1983.

Potts, Eve and Marion Morra, *Understanding Your Immune System*. New York: Avon Books, 1986.

Salaman, Maureen, *Nutrition, the CANCER ANSWER*. Menlo Park, CA: Statford Publishing, 1983.

Shelton, Herbert M., *Fasting Can Save Your Life*. Bridgeport, CN: Natural Hygiene Press, 1978.

Shelton, Herbert M., Dr. Susan Hazard and T.C. Fry, *The Cruel Hoax Called Herpes Genitalis!* Austin, Texas: Life Science, 1983.

Siegal, Frederick P., M.D., and Marta Siegal, M.A., New York: Grove Press, 1983.

Slaff, James I., M.D., and John K. Brubaker, *The AIDS Epidemic*. New York: Warner Books, 1985.

Tilden, J.H., M.D., *Toxemia Explained, Revised Edition*. Mokelumme Hill, California: Health Research, 1981.

Trowbridge, John Parks, M.D. and Morton Walker, M.D., *The Yeast Syndrome*. New York: Bantam

Books, 1986.

Urdang, Laurence, Editor-in-Chief, Helen Harding Swallow, Managing Editor, *Mosby's Medical & Nursing Dictionary*. Saint Louis, Missouri: The C. V. Mosby Company, 1983.

Walford, Roy L., M.D., *The 120 Year Diet*. New York: Simon and Schuster, 1986.

"Facts About AIDS," U.S. Department of Health and Human Services, Public Health Service, HHS Publication No. (FDA) 86–1130.